The Toke Book!
*Maximizing the Benefits
of Medical Marijuana
Through Smoking*

Revised and Expanded 2nd Edition

by

Dr. Jeff S. Gauer

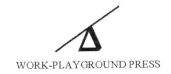

WORK-PLAYGROUND PRESS

Copyright © 2011-12 by Jeffrey S. Gauer

Cover design by Pamela Trush (www.delaney-designs.com)

All rights reserved. No part of this book may be used or reproduced in any manner whatsoever without written permission except in the case of brief quotations embodied in critical articles and reviews. For information, please contact Work-Playground Press, 1202 Glen Haven Point, Colorado Springs, CO 80907 USA.

For information on additional services, including special pricing on quantity purchases, please contact:

Work-Playground Press
Http://www.workplayground.com
E-mail: info@workplayground.com

First Printing, Jan 2012; Second Printing, Sept 2012; Third Printing, Nov 2012
Printed in the United States of America

Publisher's Cataloging-in-Publication

Gauer, Jeff S.
    The toke book! : maximizing the benefits of medical marijuana through smoking / by Jeff S. Gauer.— revised and expanded 2nd edition
    p. cm.
    Includes bibliographical references and index.
    LCCN 2012914228
    ISBN-13: 978-0-9721187-4-3
    ISBN-10: 0972118748

    1. Marijuana--Therapeutic use. 2. Cannabis--Therapeutic use.   I. Title.

RM666.C266G38 2012   615.7827
                              QBI11-600211

Foreword

Since 1995, 18 states and the District of Columbia have passed laws making marijuana medically available to seriously ill people who have the approval of their physicians. As an increasing number of patients turn to medical marijuana for pain management, Dr. Gauer's book is a useful resource for the novice medical marijuana patient. While many doctors recommend vaporizers for giving users the fast action of inhaled cannabinoids without most of the unwanted irritants, this book presents patients with additional information they'll need to start reaping the benefits of medical marijuana.

Rob Kampia
Executive Director and Co-Founder
The Marijuana Policy Project

The Toke Book! Maximizing the Benefits of Medical Marijuana through Smoking is a useful aid for the increasing numbers of marijuana naive individuals who are turning to marijuana for its incredible health benefits. While I think medibles are best under most circumstances, I particularly like the book's emphasis on a multidisciplinary approach to pain management. All life's phenomena are holistic and they emerge from the reality that the whole is greater than the sum of its parts.

Dr. Robert Melamede
Cannabinoid Biologist
Assoc. Prof. and Chairman (ret.)
Biology Dept., University of Colorado

Dedication

For pain sufferers everywhere who persevere through each day. Like my acquaintance E., who is a daily inspiration with her cheerful personality, tenacious work ethic, and exceptional parenting, all despite her chronic pain.

Other Books by Jeff Gauer

Work Can Be a Playground, Not a Prison (Basic Edition): How to Make Work Fun Again. (www.workplayground.com)

Work Can Be a Playground, Not a Prison (Professional Edition): Creating Positive Growth in Your Physical and Emotional Work Environment. (www.workplayground.com)

Gallaudet Exposed: How the World's Largest Deaf University Encourages Prejudice, Cruelty, Discrimination, and Incompetence.(www.gallaudetexposed.com)

Pain at Work: The Invisible Epidemic of Chronic Pain in America, and What We Can Do to Keep Talent in the Workplace. (www.painatwork.com)

Coming in summer '13:

S.T.R.O.N.G.E.R. Managing: Using Proven Fitness Principles to Empower Your Workforce

Author's Note

In a few years, I will reach a birthday reminding me that I have been in severe pain for fully half of my life. Pain is something I could never get used to, and pain is certainly nothing to ignore. While fighting my battle against pain, I have seen doctors all over the world and I have attempted most of the medical and holistic treatments available.

When my body screamed for more immediate pain relief, I was referred to try medical marijuana (MMJ). Only my use of MMJ, I am certain, has made it possible for me to be here today writing this book.

This manual is a collection of my research, inquiries and thoughts. As well as having Mr. Kampia's foreword, this edition also contains additional content that I hope will be useful to you. As promptly as I could I updated this text per the 2012 general election, in which voters in Washington state and Colorado, most notably, passed resolutions to legalize marijuana for recreational use. If I have made any errors, they are my own and I will try to correct them in the 3rd edition.

Thank you to all who contributed to this book, especially

- Rob Kampia, for his outstanding contribution with his foreword
- Tom Baran, who first suggested I look into MMJ
- Mom, who bought me my first MMJ and vaporizer
- Dr. Bob, for his positive support and review of my first edition
- Mona, my Strawberry, my first MMJ tutor, and my best friend for four years
- Ben, the talented owner of Grow Life, who encouraged me to share my lessons with MMJ community
- The helpful and always friendly staff at Stag Tobacconist
- Rich at A Wellness Center, for educating me about cannabis caviar
- Suzanne, my amazingly intuitive and skilled Pilates coach
- Charlene, who has always been my advocate in every way
- My little Laura, whose patience, laughter and love give me reason to smile.

Keep in mind that I was baked the whole time I wrote this book ☺. The advice in this manual is no substitute for (a) individual medical advice from your physician; or (b) individual legal advice from your attorney. Please use your MMJ responsibly and…

Enjoy!

Jeff

Table of Contents

Introduction		11
Chapter 1	Why MMJ?	17
Chapter 2	What is Pain?	27
Chapter 3	Before You Smoke	43
Chapter 4	Getting Started	49
Chapter 5	Smoking Tips and Tricks	79
Chapter 6	Conclusion	95
Glossary of Key Terms		97
Bibliography		111
End Notes		121
Appendix	Pain Information Resources	125
Subject Index		127
About the Author		129

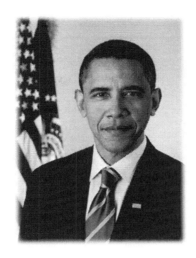

*When I was a kid I inhaled frequently.
That was the point.*

– US President Barack Obama

Introduction

Growing up in the '70s and '80s, there was hardly a time that I was *not* exposed to marijuana. In college, although marijuana was easy to find I avoided even trying pot for fear of losing my Army ROTC scholarship. So many adults in my generation experimented with weed that when I had my pre-commissioning Army physical exam, the doctor asked me, "Have you ever tried marijuana?" After I truthfully answered, "No, Sir. Never," the doctor responded, "No, really. You can tell me if you've tried it."

Even after my military service, I remained averse to trying drugs for religious reasons.[a] I've been to Amsterdam three times but never went in a "coffee shop."[b] Not wanting to encourage cigarette smoking, while in graduate school I even turned down a request to broker the sale of one million packs of cigarettes to Russia (which would have net me a six figure commission). It was not until 18 years after my

---

[a] I served as a Christian full-time missionary in Russia from 1991-92.
[b] Starting 2012, Amsterdam marijuana-dispensing coffee shops will close to tourists and be open only to Dutch citizens.

chronic pain started and I had exhausted every medical approach to relieving my back pain (including weekly epidural injections) did I consider using medical marijuana (MMJ). With my widespread pain overriding the stigma of pot smoking, plus the availability of MMJ in my state of residence (Colorado[c]), I decided to try the natural approach with weed in order to manage my pain while reducing my dependency on prescription pharmaceuticals. When I could barely move or function because of my pain, I put aside my prejudices about weed and took my medical records to a dispensary where I obtained my medical marijuana id card and made my first purchase of MMJ.

How Harmful is Marijuana?

MMJ opponents attempt to tie legal marijuana use to increased risk of crime. Researchers in California, however, examined 95 different areas in the Sacramento area. Their conclusion: there was no evidence that neighborhoods with a higher density of medical marijuana dispensaries had higher rates of violent crime or property crime than other neighborhoods.[1]

The fight against marijuana was born from economic and political agendas. Rather than consider opinions, let us look instead at the science.

> ➢ In a study published by the prestigious medical journal *The Lancet*, marijuana (Cannabis) is ranked one of the least harmful of all drugs.[2]

> ➢ Based on his study presented at the 2006 American Thoracic Society International Conference, Dr. Donald Tashkin reported:
>
>> We hypothesized that there would be a positive association between marijuana use and lung cancer, and that the association would be more positive with heavier use. What we found instead was no association at all, and even a suggestion of some protective effect.[3]

---

[c] The State of Colorado has 998 registered MMJ dispensaries, which is rumored to be more than Colorado has McDonald's restaurants.

The chart[4] below summarizes research that shows that marijuana is both less addictive and less physically harmful than alcohol and many other substances.

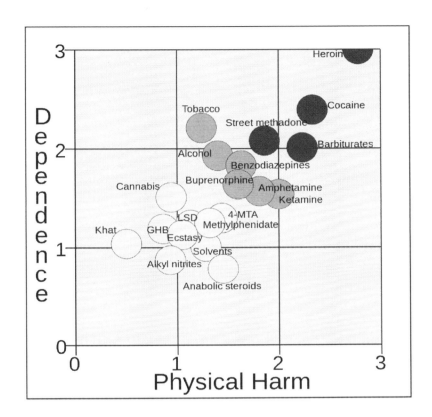

Where is MMJ Legal?

As of this printing, MMJ can be legally bought and used in the following states:

Alaska	Arizona	California
Colorado	Connecticut	DC
Delaware	Hawaii	Maine
Massachusetts	Michigan	Montana
Nevada	New Jersey	New Mexico
Oregon	Rhode Island	Vermont
Washington		

Reciprocity exists in Arizona, Delaware, Maine, Michigan, Montana and Rhode Island. If you have a valid MMJ registry (id) card issued in one of these six states, you are allowed to purchase MMJ in the other five states with reciprocity.[d] Oregon is the only state that permits out-of-state residents to apply for and receive an Oregon MMID card.[5,e]

Arizona, California, Colorado, Nevada, New Jersey, New Mexico, Maine, Oregon, Rhode Island, Montana, and Michigan are currently the only states to utilize dispensaries to sell medical cannabis. But MMJ is on the way to becoming a mainstream herbal treatment across America. In 2009, *The London Times*[6] reported:

> Across California there are an estimated 2,100 dispensaries, co-operatives, wellness clinics, and taxi delivery services in the sector known as "cannabusiness". That is more than all the Starbucks, McDonald's, and 7-Eleven outlets in the state put together.

To appreciate need for all of us to learn the benefits of MMJ for ourselves, our friends, and our family, look at the phenomenal growth in registered MMJ users in recent years:

	2004	2008	2012
Number of registered MMJ patients in Colorado[7,8]	512	4,720	96,709
Annual increase		922%	2048%

---

[d] Before going to any state where MMJ reciprocity exists, double-check yourself by calling the state's Department of Health.
[e] According to the Oregon Health Authority, nearly 600 out-of-staters have traveled to Oregon to get and use their MMID card in Oregon.

In the 2012 general election, both Washington state and Colorado passed measures that would (a) legalize the sale of marijuana to adults without the need for a doctor's prescription; and (b) reduce penalties for possession of marijuana. The same election cycle, newly elected Oregon Attorney General Ellen Rosenblum announced that she would make marijuana enforcement a low priority.[9]

In addition to the 19 states that have some form of legalized MMJ, the following 7 states currently have pending legislation to legalize MMJ:

>   Arkansas   Illinois   Missouri
>   New Hampshire   New York   Ohio
>   Pennsylvania[f]

Maryland allows for reduced penalties if cannabis use has a medical basis.[10] In 2001, Maryland passed legislation that removes fines and criminal penalties for citizens who successfully raise an 'affirmative defense' in court establishing that they possessed limited amounts (one ounce or less) of marijuana for medical purposes. Citizens who cultivate cannabis or who possess larger amounts of marijuana may still raise an affirmative defense at trial and, if successful, will have their sentence mitigated.[11] In 2003 Maryland passed a medical marijuana affirmative defense, which requires the court to consider a defendant's use of medical marijuana to be a mitigating factor in marijuana-related state prosecution. If the patient, post-arrest, successfully makes the case at trial that his or her use of marijuana is one of medical necessity, then the maximum penalty allowed by law would be a $100 fine.[12]

There is, however, still a long way to go regarding marijuana legislation. In Washington State, even though MMJ use is legal, employees can still be fired if they test positive on a drug test, despite having a doctor's prescription.[13] On a positive note, in May, 2012 a marijuana blood limit for drivers was rejected for a third time in Colorado.

---

[f] Pennsylvania's proposal contains a reciprocity provision.

The Purpose of This Book

Being a new MMJ user as well as a non-smoker, I probably made every mistake possible and went through a heck of a few years of trial and error until I figured out how to maximize the positive benefits of MMJ use. My primary purpose in writing this book is to help MMJ smokers avoid some of the mistakes I made and be able to get the most out of their MMJ.

This book is for new smokers of MMJ. If you want to prepare your own *medibles*, for example, there are plenty of good books out there so we will not get into non-smoking approaches in this manual. If you have already tried edibles and drinks containing MMJ, however, and they haven't worked for you, then give smoking a try.

Neither is this manual able to cover the complex art of growing and processing MMJ. If you are like me and purchase your MMJ from a dispensary, this book is for you.

Another reason I prefer smoking MMJ is that my expenses are lower. When I stopped making and buying medibles and drinks, my monthly cost for MMJ was 20% of what I had been spending before. So if you want to try a more cost-effective way to maximize the benefits from MMJ, read on.

In strict medical terms marijuana is far safer than many foods we commonly consume. For example, eating 10 raw potatoes can result in a toxic response. By comparison, it is physically impossible to eat enough marijuana to induce death. Marijuana in its natural form is one of the safest therapeutically active substances known to man.

— DEA Judge Francis Young

Chapter 1
Why MMJ?

You are most likely reading this book because you or a loved one suffers from a condition that you have heard can be helped by MMJ. The predominance of MMJ users are fighting some form of bodily (neuropathic) pain. I have degenerative disc disease and fibromyalgia, for example, and nothing short of an injection of Toradol gives me the immediate relief from my pain as does one good hit of MMJ.

How does MMJ work? Basically, the most well-known active ingredient in marijuana (delta-9 tetrahydrocannabinol, which is abbreviated THC) is a cannabinoid that acts on nerve cells' receptors. Some areas of the brain have many cannabinoid receptors, while other brain areas have few or none. Many cannabinoid receptors are found in the parts of the brain that influence pleasure, memory, thought, concentration, sensory and time perception, and coordinated movement.

MMJ use has been clinically shown to have positive effects for patients suffering from the following physical conditions or symptoms:

Table 1. Conditions Helped with MMJ Use	
Acquired hypothyroidism	Acute gastritis
Agoraphobia	Alcohol abuse
Alopecia Areata	AIDS related illness
Alzheimer's Disease	Anxiety
Amphetamine dependency	Amyloidosis
Amyotrophic lateral sclerosis	Amyotrophic Lateral Sclerosis (ALS)
Angina Pectoris	Ankylosis
Anorexia nervosa	Anxiety Disorders
Arteriosclerotic Heart Disease	Arthritis (Rheumatoid)
Arthropathy (Gout)	Asthma
Asthma	Atherosclerosis
Attention Deficit Hyperactivity Disorder (ADD/ADHD)	Autism/Aspergers
Autoimmune disease	Back pain/sprain
Bell's Palsy	Bipolar disorder
Bruxism	Bulimia
Brain tumor, malignant	Cachexia
Cancer, Adrenal Cortical	Cancer, Colorectal
Cancer, Endometrial	Cancer, Prostate
Cancer, Testicular	Cancer, Uterine
Carpal Tunnel Syndrome	Cerebral Palsy
Cervical Disk Disease	Cervicobrachial Syndrome
Chemotherapy	Chronic Fatigue Syndrome
Chronic pain	Chronic renal failure
Cocaine dependence	Collagen-induced arthritis
Colitis	Conjunctivitis
Constipation	Crohn's Disease
Cystic Fibrosis	Damage to spinal cord nervous tissue
Darier's Disease	Degenerative arthritis
Degenerative arthropathy	Delirium tremens
Depression	Dermatomyositis

Table 1. Conditions Helped with MMJ Use (cont'd.)	
Diabetes, Adult Onset	Diabetes, Insulin Dependent
Diabetic Neuropathy	Diabetic Peripheral Vascular Disease
Digestive diseases	Dystonia
Diarrhea	Diverticulitis
Dysthymic Disorder	Eczema
Emphysema	Endometriosis
Epidermolysis Bullosa	Epididymitis
Epilepsy	Felty's Syndrome
Fibromyalgia	Friedreich's Ataxia
Gastritis	Genital Herpes
Glaucoma	Glioblastoma Multiforme
Gliomas	Graves Disease
Headaches, cluster	Headaches, migraine
Headaches, tension	Hemophilia A
Henoch-Schonlein Purpura	Hepatitis C
Hereditary Spinal Ataxia	HIV/AIDS
HIV-associated sensory neuropathy	Hospice Patients
Huntington's Disease	Hypertension
Hyperventilation	Hypoglycemia
Impotence	Insomnia
Inflammatory autoimmune-mediated arthritis	Inflammatory Bowel Disease (IBS)
Intermittent Explosive Disorder (IED)	Intractable vomiting
Lack of appetite	Leukemia
Lipomatosis	Lou Gehrig's Disease
Lyme Disease	Lymphoma
Major depression	Malignant melanoma
Mania	Melorheostosis
Meniere's Disease	Methicillin-Resistant *Staphylococcus aureus* (MRSA)
Motion sickness	Mucopolysaccharidosis (MPS)
Multiple Sclerosis (MS)	Muscle Spasms
Muscular Dystrophy	Myeloid Leukemia
Nail-Patella Syndrome	Nausea
Nightmares	Obesity
Obsessive Compulsive Disorder (OCD)	Opiate Dependence

Table 1. Conditions Helped with MMJ Use (cont'd.)	
Osteoarthritis	Panic Disorder
Parkinson's Disease	Peripheral Neuropathy
Peritoneal Pain	Persistent Insomnia
Porphyria	Post Polio Syndrome (PPS)
Post-traumatic arthritis	Post-Traumatic Stress Disorder (PTSD)
Premenstrual syndrome (PMS)	Prostatitis
Pruritus	Psoriasis
Pulmonary Fibrosis	Quadriplegia
Radiation Therapy	Raynaud's Disease
Reiter's Syndrome	Restless Legs Syndrome (RLS)
Rosacea	Schizoaffective Disorder
Schizophrenia	Scoliosis
Sedative Dependence	Seizures
Senile Dementia	Severe nausea
Shingles (Herpes Zoster)	Sickle-cell disease
Sinusitis	Skeletal muscular spasticity
Skin tumors	Sleep apnea
Spasticity	Spinal stenosis
Sturge-Weber Syndrome (SWS)	Stuttering
Tardive Dyskinesia (TD)	Temporomandibular joint disorder (TMJ)
Tenosynovitis	Terminal illness
Thyroiditis	Tic Douloureux
Tietze's Syndrome	Tinnitus
Tobacco dependence	Tourette's Syndrome
Trichotillomania	Unintentional weight loss
Viral Hepatitis	Vomiting
Wasting Syndrome	Whiplash
Wittmaack-Ekbom's Syndrome	

Medical research seems to be catching up with what has been known for thousands of years – marijuana has many health benefits. Just in 2012, for example, a study of multiple sclerosis patients found that those who smoked cannabis had lower numbers on a spasticity scale, as well as a 50 percent decrease in pain scores.[14] In addition, advances horticultural sciences have improved the potency of cannabis, as show in the following chart compiled by data from the National Institute on Drug Abuse (NIDA):[15]

Table 2. Average Marijuana Potency by Decade	
Decade	**THC %**
1970's	1.08%
1980's	2.83%
1990's	3.76%
2000's	5.73%

Cannabinoids

THC, the most commonly recognized psychoactive in MMJ, is not the only cannabinoid in MMJ. There are six primary cannabinoids:

Cannabinoid	Description
THC Tetrahydrocannabinol (THC)	THC is the primary psychoactive component of the cannabis plant. THC eases moderate pain (analgesic) and is the cannabinoid that gives users the MMJ high.
CBD Cannabidiol (CBD)	CBD relieves convulsion, inflammation, anxiety, and nausea.[16] Research indicates that smokers of cannabis with a higher CBD/THC ratio were less likely to experience schizophrenia-like symptoms[17] (the infamous *bad trip*).
Cannabinol (CBN)	CBN is the primary product of THC degradation, and there is usually little of it in a fresh plant. CBN content increases as THC degrades in storage, and with exposure to light and air. It is only mildly psychoactive.[18]
Cannabigerol (CBG)	CBG is non-hallucinatory but increases the overall effects of cannabis. CBG has the proven ability to counteract and prevent tumors.
Tetrahydrocannabivarin (THCV)	Prevalent in certain South African and Southeast Asian strains of Cannabis, THCV increases the psychoactive effects of THC[19]. THCV is being studied for its ability to help with diabetes and with obesity.
Cannabichromene (CBC)	CBC is non-psychoactive, but has analgesic, anti-inflammatory, and antibiotic properties.

Why is it significant that MMJ can now be identifiable by specific cannabinoid? Full Spectrum Labs explains that various cannabinoids (other than THC) are beneficial:

> Even if a compound is not psychoactive, it may still have tremendous beneficial effects. Cannabinoids have numerous synergistic interactions with one another. These interactions within the body are not fully understood and do not take place with the sole administration of THC.[20]

Specialized labs can test MMJ samples (from growers, dispensaries, and MMJ dispensary clients) to identify the exact cannabinoids and ratios found in their MMJ sample. There are even home tests for cannabinoids available to purchase on-line.

Improved science allows MMJ cannabinoids to be isolated so that patients will not necessarily need to get high (from THC) to get relief of their symptoms. Patients will be able to purchase MMJ strains having only the effects they desire (e.g., stronger CBD and less THC).

As the MMJ industry grows, so has the sophistication of growers and the technology available to them. Specialized MMJ laboratories have developed ways to test strains by cannabinoid. Even without a laboratory of their own, MMJ growers can use a process called *thin-layer chromatography* (TLC) to accurately identify the cannabinoids in any strain by color, after treating the MMJ sample with a solvent system. Dispensaries using the TLC process are able to provide strains custom-grown specifically to address distinct medical conditions. The marketplace now has a variety of tools, specifically:

> The subsequent appearance on the market of diode-array or programmable variable -wavelength ultraviolet absorption detectors that can produce the absorption spectrum of a detected component, and of scanners capable of reading TLC plates in the ultraviolet and visible regions, together with the increased availability of mass spectrometers combined with gas chromatography, which are simpler for non-specialists to use, means that analytical laboratories working in cooperation with the judicial authorities in drug addiction cases can now identify cannabis samples easily, quickly and positively.[21]

The chart below shows illustrates which specific cannabinoids scientists have been able to determine help specific medical conditions. Bear in mind that cannabinoids work together in combinations that are not all yet understood.

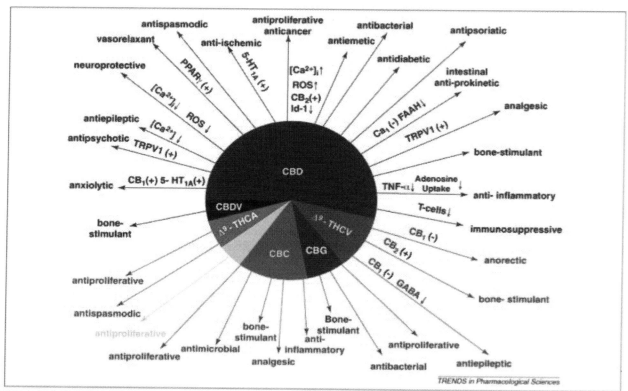

Figure 1. Pharmacological actions of non-psychotropic cannabinoids (with the indication of the proposed mechanisms of action).
Abbreviations: Δ^9-THC, Δ^9-tetrahydrocannabinol; Δ^8-THC, Δ^8-tetrahydrocannabinol; CBN, cannabinol; CBD, cannabidiol; Δ^9-THCV, Δ^9-tetrahydrocannabivarin; CBC, cannabichromene; CBG, cannabigerol; Δ^9-THCA, Δ^9-tetrahydrocannabinolic acid; CBDA, cannabidiolic acid; TRPV1, transient receptor potential vanilloid type 1; PPARγ, peroxisome proliferator-activated receptor γ; ROS, reactive oxygen species; 5-HT$_{1A}$, 5-hydroxytryptamine receptor subtype 1A; FAAH, fatty acid amide hydrolase. (+), direct or indirect activation; ↑, increase; ↓, decrease.

Reprinted from *Trends in Pharmacological Sciences, 30*(10), 515-527, Non-psychotropic plant cannabinoids: new therapeutic opportunities from an ancient herb, Angelo A. Izzo, Francesca Borrelli, Raffaele Capasso, Vincenzo Di Marzo, and Raphael Mechoulam, Copyright 2009, with permission from Elsevier.

Consolidating scientific findings from several sources[22], the table I created below lists medicinal usefulness by cannabinoid:

Cannabinoid Property	CBN	THC	CBG	THCV	CBD	CBC
protects against cancer		■	■		■	■
reduces nausea		■			■	
pain reliever	■	■			■	■
causes drowsiness	■	■				
increases appetite		■	■			
decreases appetite				■		
relieves spasms	■	■			■	
decreases seizures		■			■	■
reduces anxiety/depression		■			■	
muscle relaxant		■				
antimicrobial			■			■
aids digestion		■				
antibacterial			■		■	
antifungal			■			■
protects nervous system			■		■	■
immunosuppressive					■	
anti-diabetic					■	
improves blood circulation (vasorelaxant)		■				
minimizes organ rejection					■	
lowers blood pressure			■			
antipsychotic					■	
relieves psoriasis					■	
relieves Crohn's disease				■	■	
anti-inflammatory	■	■	■		■	■
inhibits tumor cell growth			■		■	■
bone stimulant					■	
relieves rheumatoid arthritis		■			■	
antioxidant		■			■	

With MMJ helping such a variety of problems (even hiccups!),[23] there is a good chance that smoking MMJ for one condition will help you with another. For example, smoking MMJ helps my muscle pain as well as lessens my anxiety and depression – a typical combination of symptoms experienced by fibromyalgia sufferers. According to records at the Colorado State Department of Health,[24] the most commonly reported medical conditions listed on MMID applications are:

Reported Condition	Number of Patients Reporting Condition	Percent of Patients Reporting Condition[g]
Cachexia[h]	1,191	1%
Cancer	2,510	3%
Glaucoma	1,007	1%
HIV/AIDS	617	1%
Muscle Spasms	16,532	17%
Seizures	1,615	2%
Severe Pain	90,639	94%
Severe Nausea	11,258	12%

If you are like me, your urgent priority is to lessen your pain. The next chapter may help put chronic pain in perspective and remind you that you are not alone.

---

[g] Does not add to 100% as some patients reported using medical marijuana for more than one medical condition.
[h] Weight loss, muscle atrophy, fatigue, weakness, and significant loss of appetite in someone who is not actively trying to lose weight.

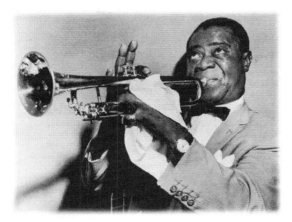

It really puzzles me to see marijuana connected with narcotics dope and all of that stuff. It is a thousand times better than whiskey. It is an assistant and a friend.

– Louis Armstrong

Chapter 2
What is Pain?[i]

Countless research studies confirm what each of us knows firsthand: **pain is far-reaching in our lives.** But did you know the following?

---

[i] Portions of this chapter are from *Pain at Work: The Invisible Epidemic of Chronic Pain in America...and What We Can Do to Keep Talent in the Workplace* by Jeff Gauer, Ph.D. (2012, Work-Playground Press – www.painatwork.com).

Ten Facts About Pain

1. Pain accounts for over 80% of all physician visits[25]

2. After seasonal colds, pain is the most common reason for visiting the doctor[26]

3. About 60-80% of active adults will experience low-back pain that is chronic (lasting more than 6 months)[27]

4. An estimated 35-50% of Americans will need medical treatment for chronic pain at some time in their lives[28]

5. Pain overrides a person's ability to concentrate and accurately recognize images[29]

6. Low back pain is the number one cause of disability in individuals 45 years and younger[30]

7. In nearly 70% of chronic pain cases, no explainable physical cause can be found[31]

8. Invisible physical disabilities affect a person more strongly than do visible disabilities[32]

9. Chronic pain is the number one cause of worker absenteeism[33]

10. Low back pain often ranks first as the cause of disability and inability to work[34]

My own 200+ page research study on chronic pain in the workplace[35] supports the following conclusions:

1. A disabling occurrence, chronic pain also affects one's mood, identity, and social behavior.

2. Pain sufferers often hide their disability from others at work (supervisors, colleagues, and subordinates), even though they are aware that their pain adversely affects their performance.

3. Having chronic pain directly and negatively affects one's work performance and long-term career success.

4. Adults suffering from chronic pain are usually not as successful in the workplace as those who do not have chronic pain, in part because people with chronic pain define success differently than those without it.

5. Pain seldom manifests in the sufferer's outward appearance, but a worker with pain hesitates to inform his or her coworkers out of fear of being stigmatized.

6. The hiding of one's pain creates a downward spiral of poor performance, which adversely affects the individual, coworkers, and the organization.

Between 25-30% of adults in industrialized nations suffer from chronic pain.[36] Financially, chronic pain represents health care costs of approximately $20 billion per year, and industry costs (e.g., disability payments, lost productivity, and training of replacement personnel) of about $80 billion annually.[37]

What is Pain?

We already intuitively know what pain is, but better understanding how our bodies process pain can prepare us with the means to cope with it.

Pain is both a physical experience (the biological state of the body) and a physiological experience (how the body functions). Pain is attributable to these material factors (e.g., a torn muscle, which is physical and physiological) as well as psychological factors (e.g. emotional frame of mind).

The cause of pain is often obscure. For example, low back pain is directly linked to a defined, organic disease only in a minority of cases.[38] A report to the Chronic Pain Panels for the Ontario Workplace Safety and Insurance Board explained, "All pain . . . is a phenomenon that affects, and is affected, by both mind and body".[39] Non-Specific Lower Back Pain (NSLBP) is defined by having neither nerve-root compression nor a serious underlying condition.[40] The NSLBP diagnosis is based on symptoms and not on "verifiable physical pathology or the presence of an anatomical lesion."[41] A 2003 study by Ehrlich instructs that

> NSLBP is neither a disease nor a diagnostic entity of any sort. The term refers to pain of variable duration in an area of the anatomy afflicted so often that it has become a paradigm of responses to external and internal stimuli.[42]

Regardless of its cause, pain affects adults' individual job performance.[43] In 2007, researchers used brain scans to demonstrate that pain overrides a person's ability to concentrate and accurately recognize images.[44]

Chronic Pain

Now is a good time to review what it means when we say that pain is *chronic*. Chronic pain (as opposed to acute pain) is a persistent, and real, neural sensation that may or may not be attributed to a past injury or evidence of bodily damage. In other words, chronic pain is pain felt over a long period of time for which no specific cause is always known.

A person with chronic pain may feel specific or generalized soreness, which can range from aching, burning, or tingling to a pain that is stabbing or breath catching. Described as a "multidimensional phenomenon involving sensory, affective, motivational, and cognitive components"[45] and a "constellation of symptoms,"[46] chronic pain can cause dizziness, nausea, overwhelming fatigue, lack of concentration, and other symptoms.

Chronic pain is typically very frustrating for sufferers as well as for their caregivers, friends, and associates. This is because chronic pain is complicated "by a hostile environment and aggravated by legal and compensation issues"[47] as well as by "heroic treatments that ultimately fail to help and may even be harmful."[48] Research proves that chronic pain limits an individual's ability and motivation to work,[49] which is pretty common sense if you have ever endured pain lasting more than a few weeks. Pain is considered to be *chronic* when it:

1. Has "no clearly identifiable cause"[50]
2. "Continues in the presence or absence of demonstrable pathology"[51]
3. Persists for longer than the 6 months the body normally needs in order to rebuild tissues.[52]

Researchers Khalsa and Stauth add the following,

> Chronic pain is not a symptom… not a warning that something is wrong …. For the most part chronic pain is a disease….Chronic pain is in the brain–usually a malfunction of the nervous system.[53]

Chronic pain is, by definition, expected not to diminish for the sufferer[54]. Chronic pain disrupts sleep and normal living, and actually ceases to serve the body's protective function.[55] Pain neurons change the body's reaction to pain, actually causing previously noninjured tissue to react like injured tissue[56] and making each painful episode worse than the last.[57]

In addition to having longer-lasting and intensified pain, chronic pain sufferers have been found to exhibit self-destructive behaviors such as *fear avoidance*[58], *workers' compensation syndrome*,[59] and *disability syndrome*.[60,j]

---

[j] These three work-related syndromes are covered in detail in Chapter 6 (Returning to Work) of my fourth book, *Pain at Work: The Invisible Epidemic of Chronic Pain in America…and What We Can Do to Keep Talent in the Workplace* (2012, Work-Playground Press – www.painatwork.com).

Low Back Pain

The most common type of chronic pain is *nonspecific low-back pain* (NSLBP), which affects about 60-80% of the active adult population at some point over the course of a lifetime, and accounts for over 90% of all low-back pain cases.[61] Low-back pain ranks "often first as a cause of disability and inability to work, as an interference with the quality of life, and as a reason for medical consultation."[62] Low back pain is the number one cause of disability in workers 45 years old and younger.[63] In any given year, 40% of adults suffer from low-back pain more than 1 day in the previous 12 days, and 15% of low-back-pain sufferers are in pain throughout the year.[64]

Pain and Stress

As far as I am concerned, you cannot have a discussion about pain without including the powerful impact of stress. Much has been studied about the interrelationships of biological, psychological, and sociological factors influencing the onset, intensity, and alleviation of chronic pain among workers.[65] The six models discussed in this section illustrate the chronological development of multidisciplinary views regarding individuals, their environments, and their pain.

Stress is a frequent player in the onset and development of chronic pain. Researchers have explained that, depending on their personal capability to deal with stress, workers respond differently to the stresses imposed by their jobs.[66] The earliest research on stress reactions to environment was Cannon's 1929 discovery of organisms' physiological response to stress (the *fight or flight phenomenon*).[67]

Seven years later, Selye developed this concept into an explanation of how stressors affect an organism's response:

Three-Stage General Adaptation Syndrome

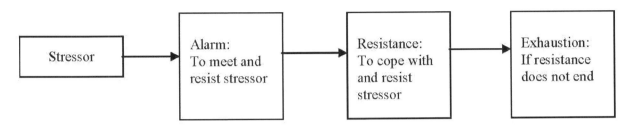

From "A syndrome produced by diverse nocuous agents," by H. Selye, 1936, *Nature, 138,* p. 32. Copyright 1936 by Macmillan Magazines. Reprinted with permission.

In terms of chronic pain, we can follow Selye's model from left to right in three stages:

- Stage 1: Pain (*stressor*) materializes (*alarm*)

- Stage 2: The sufferer attempts to cope (*resistance*) through medical treatment[68], as well as by utilizing social support systems.[69]

- Stage 3: When the pain does not subside the sufferer becomes more dispirited and disabled (*exhaustion*).[70] Bear in mind that, because narcotics and opioid analgesics are generally the first line of treatment for the symptoms of chronic pain,[71] the exhaustion factor is made worse by the medications taken.

In 1975, Selye developed a model dividing stress into *eustress* and *distress*.[72] Where stress enhances an individual's physical or mental abilities (such as through strength training or challenging work), it may be considered *eustress*. Persistent stress that is not resolved through coping or adaptation, deemed *distress*, may lead to anxiety or withdrawal (depression) behavior. The difference between experiences that result in *eustress* and those that result in *distress* is determined by the disparity between an experience (real or imagined) and personal expectations, and resources to cope with the stress.[73]

> *Every stress leaves an indelible scar, and the organism pays for its survival after a stressful situation by becoming a little older.*
>
> **- Hans Selye**

Following the lead of Cannon[74] and Selye,[75] other researchers[76] expanded on these concepts, showing how extended stress produces irreversible exhaustion. The years 1978-79 saw the publication of two new frameworks dealing with the individual's ability to cope with being in a stressful environment over time.

The Person-Environment Fit Model (below) illustrates how a disconnect between an employee and her work environment results in physical strain and eventual illness.[77] More precisely, the more realistically an individual perceives her situation, the better she will be able to deal with her situation. If an employee's assessment of herself and her workplace are accurate (see left side), then coping satisfies her needs and she experiences little or no strain. If, however, the employee perceives her workplace and herself in an unrealistic manner, then her defense mechanisms kick in. The immediate result is anxiety (strain); the long-term result is a weakened physical condition (illness).

Person-Environment Fit Model

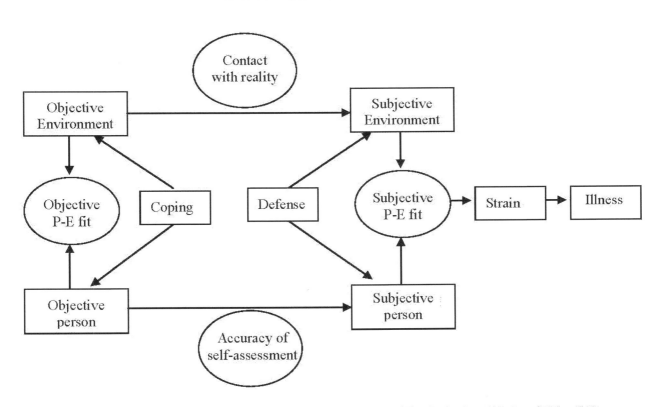

From *Stress at Work* (p. 175), by C. L. Cooper and R. Payne (Eds.), 1978, Chichester, NY: John Wiley & Sons. Copyright 1978 by the publisher. Reprinted with permission.

Moving from the broader model of the person/ environment fit, the Job Strain Model[78] (below) illustrates that when a worker's job has high demands yet provides him little decision control, his stress is increased.

Job Strain Model

		Job Demands	
		Low	High
Decision Control — High		Low strain	Active
Decision Control — Low		Passive	High strain

From "Job demands, job decision latitude, and mental strain: Implications for job redesign" (p. 286), by R. Karasek, 1979, *Administration Science Quarterly, 24,* 285-308. Copyright 1979 by The Johnson School at Cornell University. Reprinted with permission.

In 1992 was published what I consider to be the clearest depiction of chronic pain's multifaceted influences. The Biopsychosocial Model[79] (next page) explains how the biological, psychological, and social factors of chronic pain sufferers interact; and that this interaction influences the onset and progression of disease.

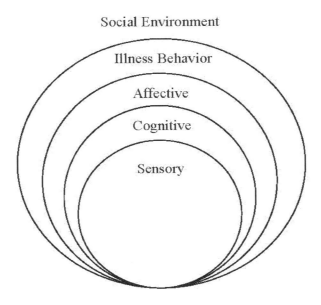

From "Biopsychosocial analysis of low back pain" (p. 523), by G. Waddell, 1992, in M. Nordin & T. L. Visher (Eds.), *Bailiere's clinical rheumatology, common low back pain: Prevention of chronicity* (pp. 523-557). London: Bailiere Tindall. Copyright 1992 by Elsevier. Reprinted with permission.

To clarify the biopsychosocial model, keep in mind that *affective* behavior is synonymous with *emotional*. We can explain the model in narrative form as follows,

1. Our senses pick up on our social environment (sensory/biological)
2. Our brain works to make sense of our social environment (cognitive/mental)
3. Based on our character and experiences—plus the input received through our five senses—we interpret our social environment in terms of our feelings (affective)
4. If our body and mind are unable to cope with the combination of biological, emotional, and social stimuli, we become incapacitated (illness behavior).

The biopsychosocial model is supported by other research studies, four conclusions of which follow:

1. Emotions impact the perception and intensity of pain[80]
2. Pain differs from person to person, and culture to culture[81]
3. Psychosocial factors more strongly influence the continuation of chronic pain symptoms than do biological or physical factors[82]
4. The nature of a person's pain often has little to do with his or her objective physical condition, but is based rather on the individual's response to the pain.[83]

One year after the biopsychosocial model was published, a team of researchers[84] discovered that stress (from psychosocial factors and individual characteristics) contributes to musculoskeletal disease and chronic symptoms. The Model of Stress and Musculoskeletal Disease (below) depicts the interaction of psychosocial, environmental and personal/individual factors, which lead to chronic symptoms, such as pain, absenteeism, medicine use, and/or disability.

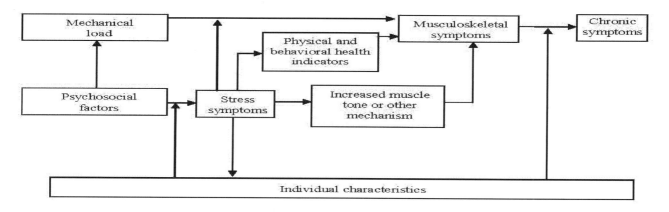

From "Psychosocial factors at work and musculoskeletal disease" (p. 297), by P. M. Bongers, C. R. deWinter, M. A. Kompier, & V. H. Hildebrandt, 1993, *Scandinavian Journal of Work and Environment Health, 19*(5), 297-312. Copyright 1993 by the publisher. Reprinted with permission.

Also in the 1990's, researchers[85] made the connection between lower back pain and four risk factors. As seen below, there is a continuous, dynamic cycle of factors that affect the worker:

Risk Factors in Lower Back Pain

```
              Organizational
                 factors
                    │
         ┌──────────┼──────────┐
         │          ▼          │
    Physical     Worker    Individual
    workload    ───────    factors
         │          ▲          │
         └──────────┼──────────┘
                    │
              Psychological
                 factors
```

From "Challenges in assessing risk factors in epidemiologic studies on back disorders" (p. 143), by Burdorf et al., 1997. *American Journal of Industrial Medicine,* 32(2), p. 143. Copyright 1997 by Wiley-Liss, Inc. a subsidiary of John Wiley & Sons, Inc. Reprinted with permission.

For the chronic pain sufferer, pain (*individual factors*) affects their mood and identity,[86] and feelings (*psychological factors*) affect behavior.[87] With chronic pain, the constant physical and psychosocial factors exacerbate the pain[88] as well as increase the negative impact of external stress (*organizational)* factors, leading to a downward spiral for the sufferer.[89]

If you would like to learn more about managing stress and interpersonal challenges in the workplace, consider reading my earlier books (see www.workplayground.com):

> ➢ Work Can Be a Playground, Not a Prison (Professional Edition): *Creating Positive Growth in Your Physical and Emotional Work Environment*

> ➢ Work Can Be a Playground, Not a Prison (Basic Edition): *How to Make Work Fun Again*

Pain vs. Sleep

Chronic pain sufferers frequently lack the delta level sleep required to restore the neurotransmitters in their muscles. Muscle pain combined with sleep deprivation results in a brutal downward spiral for the afflicted person. The next two graphics illustrate the pain-exhaustion cycle:

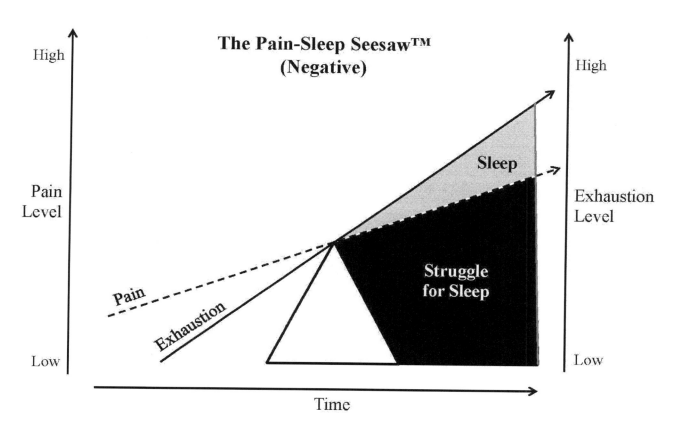

© 2012 Jeff S. Gauer. All rights reserved.

Depicted above, the sensations of pain and exhaustion for chronic pain sufferers ebb and flow, each on its own linear spectrum. Rarely does a pain sufferer feel not tired <u>and</u> not sore, but she fights to reduce her pain and exhaustion even though as one increases so does the other. The problem arises when her pain exceeds her exhaustion[k]. The sufferer is often forced to rely on medication or other sedatives in

---
[k] Millions of chronic pain sufferers live like this 24/7.

order to overcome enough pain to let her tiredness take over. Such forced sleep, however, is not as restful as natural sleep. Pain sufferers frequently:

1. Build up a tolerance to sedatives and need to take more and more every day in order to maintain their medications' efficacy.

2. Wake up groggy and sore from each drugged sleep.

A more favorable pain-sleep scenario is shown below:

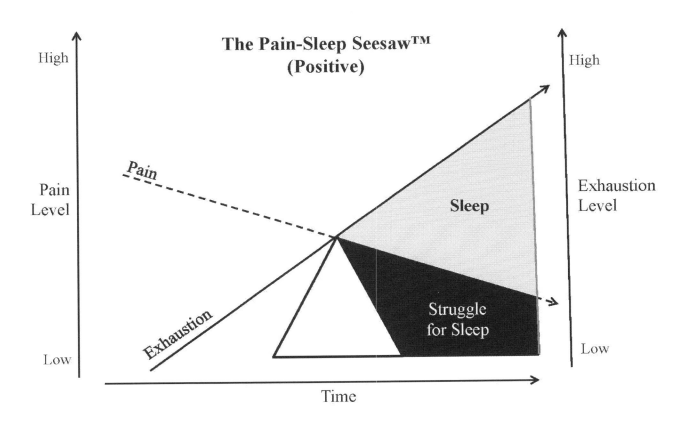

© 2012 Jeff S. Gauer. All rights reserved.

As discussed in Chapter 1, smoking medical marijuana helps sufferers lower their pain, stress, and anxiety, thus making it easier to achieve natural, restorative sleep. In this *positive* Pain-Sleep Seesaw we see a healthier, more natural progression. As a person becomes increasingly tired through his day, he reaches the point where he is exhausted enough in order to sleep but not in too much pain to be kept awake. Tiredness in this scenario far exceeds the person's pain, which is a great thing for the sleep deprived.

Conclusion

The research studies reviewed in this chapter show definitively that chronic pain is not exclusively a physical problem. Chronic pain can be brought on—and certainly can be made worse—by psychological, social, and other environmental factors. Building upon these developments, researchers[90] have proven that cognitive-behavioral approaches to chronic pain and pain programs are useful in uncovering the dynamics of chronic pain sufferers' conditions. When treated with a multidisciplinary approach, those with chronic pain have been able to heighten their awareness of the biopsychosocial processes that contribute to their disease, and use this knowledge to take steps toward mitigating their pain experience.[91]

If you would like to discover more about coping with chronic pain in the workplace, I expect to release my next book in January '13:

>Pain at Work: *The Invisible Epidemic of Chronic Pain in America, and What We Can Do to Keep Talent in the Workplace* (www.painatwork.com).

Fortunately, MMJ has been clinically proven to help alleviate physical pain as well as reduce stress. Whereas increased anxiety and pain can become a downward spiral feeding off each other, MMJ can stop and reverse this spiral and give your body and your mind a break. Even your smoking routine (of preparing your herb, smoking, and cleaning your receptacle) can be calming and help with your stress.

Now that we know a little more about MMJ and pain, the next chapter will cover the various options available for smoking your MMJ.

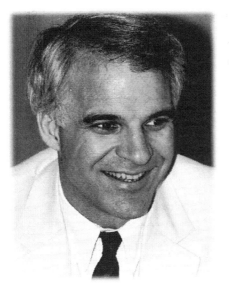

I used to smoke marijuana. But I'll tell you something: I would only smoke it in the late evening. Oh, occasionally the early evening, but usually the late evening - or the mid-evening. Just the early evening, midevening and late evening. Occasionally, early afternoon, early midafternoon, or perhaps the late-midafternoon. Oh, sometimes the early-mid-late-early morning. . . . But never at dusk.

– Steve Martin

Chapter 3
Before You Smoke

You now have your MMJ and everything you decided you needed to smoke. But before you light up the first time, here is some advice.

Have a drink handy. Smoking MMJ will dry your mouth out, and many people like having a fruit-flavored drink like Gatorade® handy, but water works too.

Be sitting down when you smoke. Be careful standing up after smoking. Before standing up, make sure you are steady and not lightheaded. Smoking strongly raises your heart rate and your blood pressure. If you stand up too fast, your blood pressure may drop significantly (I've passed out three times myself). Likewise, it is not wise to smoke MMJ and get in a hot tub – unless you want to risk giving yourself a stroke or heart attack. Holding your breath to maximum will likewise increase your heart rate and blood pressure, which is why you get a better toke when you really hold your breath.

Presuming you are ready to light up, and have all your supplies ready, the only thing to do next is train your lungs. Do not try to inhale deeply at first. Inhale just enough MMJ (letting outside air in through the sides of your mouth) to feel the effect. Gradually your lungs will become used to smoking and you will be able to take deeper and longer hits. Even experienced MMJ smokers often leave enough room in their lungs during a hit to be able to follow their toke with a gulp of fresh air. Ironically, by the time you are an experienced smoker you will have to smoke more MMJ anyway if you want to reach the same high as you did as a new smoker.

As you inhale from your joint, vaporizer or pipe, remember to hold your breath. I would prefer to hold my breath longer (8-12 seconds) with less smoke in my lungs than try to gulp a lungful of smoke and fight to keep from coughing. Until you are comfortable with MMJ smoking and know how it affects you:

- Exhale your toke if you feel lightheaded or dizzy while holding the smoke in your lungs

- To see how your body reacts and to prevent getting too high (or a bad trip, which is even worse), always wait 2-3 minutes after each toke before you take another hit. Some strains can sneak up on you after you have already exhaled; some effects can even hit you after a few minutes. It also is a good idea to give your lungs a break between tokes.

What Does a High Feel Like?

Everyone has different tolerances, and some of us react unusually to medications[1]. In general, however, most people feel some (or all) of the following sensations when they smoke MMJ:

- Immediate pain relief
- Tingling up and down your body
- Lightness, like your head is a balloon[m]
- Dizziness
- Heavy eyes and relaxed muscles
- Sense of calm and well-being, sometimes euphoric
- Dry mouth
- Short-term memory loss
- Food cravings or increased appetite
- Decreased motor coordination
- Intense concentration or focus

After taking a hit of MMJ and exhaling, I find it comfortable to take a deep breath of fresh air and hold it for two seconds before exhaling again. This seems to lessen my nausea and dizziness immediately after a toke.

Bad Trips[n]

Have a friend with you when you smoke, especially when you are new to MMJ. It is possible to consume too much MMJ. Some people can experience "a bad trip" when after smoking MMJ the person feels overwhelming paranoia and panic. A friend smoking MMJ with me, for example, became afraid she could not leave the room and desperately needed repeated assurance from me that she could.

A bad trip usually involves having an uneasy, anxious feeling; sometimes the room spins, and you might even have slight hallucinations. Don't worry! No one has ever died from marijuana. Relax! Try to sit perfectly still and focus on something

---

[1] My first wife, for example, would drink a cup of coffee if she couldn't sleep. Caffeine actually had the reverse effect on her, making her drowsy.

[m] Sometimes a throbbing headache accompanies a strong Sativa (head) high.

[n] Portions of this section included by generous permission of Northern Lights Natural Rx (http://nlnaturalrx.com).

external (TV, radio, book). Concentrate on slowing your breathing and your heart rate. Eventually the effects will wear off.

It never hurts to have a friend nearby to talk you through a potential bad trip, especially if you are new to MMJ. Turning on a favorite TV show or movie[o] to distract yourself can also help you get through a bad trip. If the feeling you are experiencing is too uncomfortable you can take activated charcoal. Activated charcoal can be found in pill form in health food stores; it will help absorb the THC to minimize the negative effects you feel.

If you have a bad trip, try switching MMJ strains.

> Regardless of how you smoke MMJ, the <u>deeper</u> you inhale and the <u>longer</u> you hold your breath before exhaling, the stronger the MMJ effect you will feel.

Important Closing Thoughts

Do not stop taking your existing medications without discussing with your doctor first! While still recovering from spinal fusion surgery in 2009, I was using morphine patches for pain when I first got my MMJ card. The owner of the dispensary I visited told me that MMJ would be an easy substitute for morphine and that I could just go "cold turkey." After suffering through three days of serious morphine withdrawal – *while* also trying to get used to the new sensation of smoking MMJ – I put my morphine patch back on. I decreased the patch size a little bit each day until I was free from the morphine after about two weeks.

---

[o] A great way to enjoy a high is by listening to Pink Floyd's "Dark Side of the Moon" while watching "The Wizard of Oz" muted (start Floyd at the 3rd roar of the MGM lion).

If you struggle paying for your MMJ, check with your state's Department of Health about any financial assistance programs, for example:

➢ Colorado has an organization called Coloradans 4 Cannabis (www.C4CPR.org) which provides per month one donated 1/8 gram of MMJ and reduced pricing ($25) for additional 1/8 grams purchased from contributing MMJ dispensaries.

➢ The Medical Marijuana Assistance Program of America (MMAPA – www.mmapa.us) services Arizona, Colorado, Maine, Massachusetts, New Jersey, and Vermont. Each MMAPA member is allotted one ounce of cannabis per month at the discounted price (30-50%), based on the applicant's income level, household size, and in which state and federal programs they are already enrolled. Veterans receive an automatic 50% discount with proof of veteran status (form DD 214).

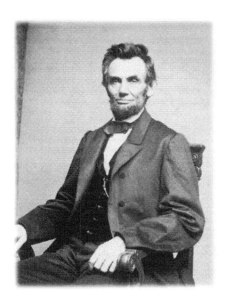

Two of my favorite things are sitting on my front porch smoking a pipe of sweet hemp, and playing my Hohner harmonica.

– US President Abraham Lincoln

Chapter 4
Getting Started

So you have decided to give MMJ a try. In this chapter, we will cover the steps you can take to obtaining, preparing, and smoking your MMJ. First, however, let us take a quick look at what part of the marijuana plant you will be smoking, and for which uses other plant parts can be applied.

Anatomy of a Marijuana Plant

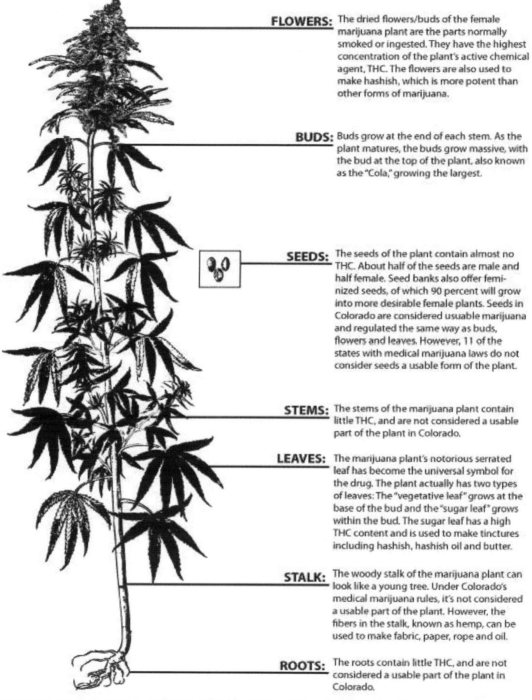

FLOWERS: The dried flowers/buds of the female marijuana plant are the parts normally smoked or ingested. They have the highest concentration of the plant's active chemical agent, THC. The flowers are also used to make hashish, which is more potent than other forms of marijuana.

BUDS: Buds grow at the end of each stem. As the plant matures, the buds grow massive, with the bud at the top of the plant, also known as the "Cola," growing the largest.

SEEDS: The seeds of the plant contain almost no THC. About half of the seeds are male and half female. Seed banks also offer feminized seeds, of which 90 percent will grow into more desirable female plants. Seeds in Colorado are considered usuable marijuana and regulated the same way as buds, flowers and leaves. However, 11 of the states with medical marijuana laws do not consider seeds a usable form of the plant.

STEMS: The stems of the marijuana plant contain little THC, and are not considered a usable part of the plant in Colorado.

LEAVES: The marijuana plant's notorious serrated leaf has become the universal symbol for the drug. The plant actually has two types of leaves: The "vegetative leaf" grows at the base of the bud and the "sugar leaf" grows within the bud. The sugar leaf has a high THC content and is used to make tinctures including hashish, hashish oil and butter.

STALK: The woody stalk of the marijuana plant can look like a young tree. Under Colorado's medical marijuana rules, it's not considered a usable part of the plant. However, the fibers in the stalk, known as hemp, can be used to make fabric, paper, rope and oil.

ROOTS: The roots contain little THC, and are not considered a usable part of the plant in Colorado.

Sources: Leonhart Fuchs, "Das Kräuterbuch," 1543; Otto Wilhelm Thomé, "Flora von Deutschland, Österreich und der Schweiz," 1885; Flickr user Bob Doran shared with a Creative Commons attribution license; Kevin Bonsor for Discovery Health, "How Marijuana Works"

Selecting a Dispensary

The first thing you will need to do is check if your state has a legalized MMJ program (see p. 13) and get yourself a medical marijuana id (registry) card. Contact information for MMJ dispensaries is easily found on the Internet. If you are in a state like Colorado you may simply find a dispensary off the road (look for the green plus sign). Most dispensaries have (or can refer you to) a licensed physician who will screen you for your MMJ card and complete the necessary paperwork with you.

Bring with you to your doctor's appointment a copy of your medical records and proof of identification. The more evidence of your condition and symptoms, the easier it will be for the MMJ-friendly physician to sign off on your MMJ card application. Be prepared to pay $150-350 for the physician visit,[p] after which you should be given a temporary MMJ card (your permanent one-year MMJ card should arrive in your mailbox in about a month).

Once you have your temporary MMJ card, you have the legal right to purchase MMJ at any dispensary in your state of residence (and reciprocating states, if any – see p.13). First time MMID applicants with a temporary MMJ card need to show proof that they mailed their state application, as well as show copies of their physician certification and state application, before dispensaries are permitted to sell MMJ to them. The Colorado Department of Health (CODOH) maintains a website of denied MMJ applications, so Colorado dispensaries will sell to temporary MMID holders as long as their application number does not show "denied" on the CODOH website.

With MMJ dispensaries now outnumbering Starbucks in some states, a very real concern is finding a quality dispensary. If you do not have a personal referral to a dispensary, here are some signs of a good MMJ dispensary:

- ✓ How long have they been in business? Be wary of dispensaries that have been open for only a few months (they may not be around for long – for example, 28% of MMJ dispensaries registered in 2011 were already out of business by Jan 2012)

- ✓ Do they carry a variety of fresh strains (at least 2-3 strains each of Indica and Sativa)?

---

[p] State fee ($90 in Colorado) plus physician's fees.

- ✓ Do they grow their own strains (a requirement in some states) or purchase from a grower? Dispensaries that grown their own product not only show a vesting interest in their cannabis, their staff also tend to be more knowledgeable about the strains they sell.

I probably tried out ten different dispensaries in my home state until deciding upon one having the products, service, prices and ambience that suit me.

States have different models for assigning MMJ caregivers. In Colorado, your MMJ application has a designation for your "primary caregiver" (dispensary), but this is more of an administrative/legal detail for the dispensary's sake – to legally grow and possess MMJ, dispensaries (caregivers) must have patients assigned to them to provide MMJ. Assigning a MMJ caregiver supports your dispensary and helps your state MMJ system work. In Colorado at least,

- ➢ You are not legally required to assign a caregiver
- ➢ You can change your primary caregiver anytime you like
- ➢ You can even shop at any dispensary in your state without changing your primary caregiver

Your state Department of Health can provide the specific regulations for your state regarding caregiver assignment.

There are quite a few options for getting MMJ (actually the psychoactive elements called cannabinoids) into your body. Marijuana has been cultivated and used as far back as 8,000 BC. Usually smoked, MMJ is also available to consume as:

- Food (*medible*), such as brownies, cookies, fudge, gummy bears, bubble gum and lollipops
- Carbonated and non-carbonated drinks and shots
- Topical lotions, creams and tinctures
- THC capsules

If you, like me, have tried the non-smoking route and are unsatisfied with the effect, keep reading.

Why Smoke?

Clinical research shows that absorbing MMJ through the lungs is faster than other ways of taking in THC. The following is from an often-referenced research German study, "Pharmacokinetics and Pharmacodynamics of Cannabinoids":[92]

> The pharmacokinetics of THC vary as a function of its route of administration. Pulmonary assimilation of inhaled THC causes a maximum plasma concentration within minutes, psychotropic effects start within seconds to a few minutes, reach a maximum after 15 to 30 minutes, and taper off within 2 to 3 hours. Following oral ingestion, psychotropic effects set in with a delay of 30 to 90 minutes, reach their maximum after 2 to 3 hours and last for about 4 to 12 hours, depending on dose and specific effect.

To put it more simply, smoking MMJ starts the effect of THC almost immediately. When eating or drinking products containing MMJ, however, the THC effects begin after a half hour or more.[q] You personally need to weigh the health risks[r] of smoking against your need for immediate physical and emotional relief through smoking MMJ.

Containers

The best MMJ containers I have encountered are *pop top bottles* (shown on right). These plastic containers are air-tight and can be opened with one hand, which is handy when you are filling your pipe. The majority of MMJ dispensaries still put patients' MMJ in zip-lock plastic bags or prescription bottles (neither of which are airtight), but you can encourage your dispensary to carry pop top bottles.

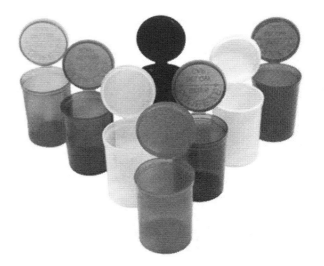

---

[q] Though the effects from oral ingestion generally last longer.
[r] It has been reported that marijuana smoke contains 3 times the amount of tar found in tobacco smoke and 50 percent more carcinogens.

Choosing a Strain

There are two principle strains of MMJ: Sativa and Indica. Your dispensary will most likely carry a variety of strains ranging from mostly Sativa to mostly Indica, plus hybrids (blends) in between. MMJ dispensary staff should be able to tell you the percent of sativa/indica in each strain they sell. You basically, then, have three categories of bud available at your dispensary:

Indica – Has strong pain relieving properties, often called a "body effect."

Sativa – Gives more of a "head high" with energetic and uplifting effects.

Hybrid – In order to capture specific desired qualities from different MMJ strains, marijuana growers will combine (usually) two different MMJ plants into one new (hybrid) strain having properties of both parent plants.

Hash

In addition to smoking tobacco and MMJ, you can also smoke MMJ extracts (with your tobacco alone, or in combination with your tobacco and bud). The most common MMJ extract sold in dispensaries is *hash*, which is a concentration of resin glands, created using natural stripping solvents such as water and ice. Below are some of the basic forms of hash that you can purchase and smoke:

- The most common form of hash is **bubble hash**. Bubble hash is named so because the names of the bags/screens used to filter the hash are bubble bags.
- Lighter colored hash (***blonde***) tends to have more of a sativa "head high"
- Darker colored hash will contain more plant matter resulting in more of an Indica (body) effect along with a strong head high.
- ***Earwax*** is a strong form of hash that is generally made using a non-natural solvent such as butane or carbon dioxide.[s]

---

[s] Creating oil and earwax using these solvents can be very dangerous and should only be attempted by professionals.

Keep an Eye Out for New MMJ Products

It seems to me that at least every couple of months, new MMJ products arrive in the marketplace. Dispensaries in California and Colorado, for example, continue to develop new ways to increase the potency of their bud. The following is a summary of three types of enhanced MMJ, listed in increasing order of potency:

1. Tossing MMJ bud in a tumbler with kief makes ***super charged*** bud.
2. MMJ bud soaked in hash oil is often called ***infused flower***.
3. ***Caviar*** is made by rolling infused flower in kief and then dried. Cannabis caviar is currently the most potent (and most expensive) form of enhanced MMJ available to MMID card holders.

Any of these enhanced forms of MMJ bud are stronger than your basic harvested and dried MMJ. You will, of course, see that the prices for these are higher. But even though enhanced MMJ is more expensive, you may find yourself spending less money overall out of your MMJ budget because you may not need to smoke as often (or as much) of enhanced MMJ.

Experiment!

Before you stock up on MMJ that might not be the most cost-effective for you, you need to determine what form(s) of MMJ works best for you. Try smoking various strains and combinations. Rather than buying ½ oz. of one strain from your dispensary, experiment with smaller amounts of multiple MMJ strains.

When you experiment, however, remember that it is critical to keep track of what works for you. If necessary, take written notes[t] to keep track of how each MMJ products/strain affects you after smoking.

Or consider a simpler approach. Based on the effect you feel after smoking each strain, respectively, organize and label your containers of various MMJ strains in a row from "the most Indica" to "the most Sativa." Storing your MMJ in such an order makes it quick and easy to select which MMJ (or combination) will relieve your specific symptoms when you need it.

---

[t] Do you really think that you will remember your thoughts the next day?!? ☺

Keep in mind, when we smoke MMJ our bodies build up resistance to its effects. You can mitigate your body's tolerance to MMJ by switching–or even just rotating among–strains every few weeks or so.

Depending on your MMJ smoking goals (see pp.16-24) the experienced staff at your dispensary can probably recommend strains for you. MMJ dispensaries sell individual pre-rolled joints as well as buds. MMJ bud is sold by weight usually starting at 1/8 oz.[u] Hash is sold by the gram, usually starting at ½ gram. Personally I purchase mostly Indica MMJ (for my pain) but I also like getting the Sativa high sometimes, so I try to keep the following MMJ in stock at home:

- ✓ ½ oz. pure Indica – split into two different strains
- ✓ ¼ oz. Sativa dominant (e.g., 70% Sativa, 30% Indica)
- ✓ 1 oz. Indica dominant (e.g., 80% Indica, 20% Sativa) – split into 2-3 different strains
- ✓ 1 gram *caviar* (or *bubble hash* or *ear wax*).

How Much MMJ Can I Buy?

Most states set MMID holders to an MMJ purchase limit (i.e. how much MMJ you can possess at one time) per person per month, usually between 1-3 oz.[v]

Seeds and Stems

When you purchase MMJ, it will usually have stems (the bud grows out of the stem). You may even occasionally find seeds with your buds.[w] What you do not want to do, however, is smoke either the seeds or the stems. Smoking MMJ seeds can give you a headache, and research indicates that smoking MMJ seeds may lower the sperm count in men.

MMJ stems do have trichomes but very little THC is on them. I will crush thin stems into my pipe but I throw away the thick branch-like stems. Stems give a harsher smoke and headaches, so I wouldn't recommend smoking only MMJ stems.

---

[u] Your dispensary may sell MMJ by the gram or 1/16th oz.
[v] California's limit is 8 oz.; Washington State's limit is 24 oz. per month.
[w] You can save these for planting yourself!

How Small Should I Grind?

When you smoke, you want maximize the surface area of the product that you are heating/burning. Here is a basic rule of thumb:

- Large grind (hand-picked) – Good for pipe smoking
- Medium grind (manual MMJ grinder) – Good for making joints or vaporizing.
- Small grind (coffee grinder) – Best for baking and cooking medibles.

Signs of Quality MMJ

When you are shopping for MMJ, the buds you buy should be green and moist, with a pungent smell. If the weed is dry and brittle, the MMJ is old and has probably been sitting around the dispensary for a few weeks (incidentally also losing its potency).

> If the weed is brown, turn it down.
> If the weed is dry, pass it by.

I wish to add one caveat to my advice above. If you are purchasing enhanced MMJ buds, these are **purposely** dried as part of the infusion process. So do not reject cannabis caviar just because it is dry – caviar and other enhanced bud (e.g., super charged, and infused flower) should appear that way.

If you get a severe headache and/or nausea immediately after smoking a bowl of MMJ (often the feeling can last for hours), do not automatically assume that it is your fault. Smokers can suffer severe side effects from MMJ that is not adequately *flushed* by the grower. Flushing is when the grower uses water and special hydroponic formulas to purge salts and chemicals from the cannabis plants and soil prior to harvesting. If MMJ is harvested without being properly flushed, dried and cured, you might see either or both of the following signs:

- Your MMJ is difficult to ignite and keep lit
- Your MMJ burns to dark ash instead of white, fluffy ash

Either of these two signals may warn you that fertilizer salts, chemicals and/or other pollutants may have been retained in the MMJ bud that you are smoking.

In short, if you get an immediate headache or nausea after smoking your MMJ, it might be the weed grower's fault for not sufficiently flushing his crop. Try buying some MMJ from a different dispensary and see if your headaches go away.

Smoking Options

THC is absorbed quickly through the lungs by smoking MMJ and there are three basic methods to accomplish this:

1. Joint
2. Vaporizer
3. Pipe

Joint

A joint is basically an MMJ cigarette. To make a joint, you will need the following:

- A gram or less of crushed MMJ
- Cigarette (rolling) paper
- Some cigarette tobacco (optional)
- Rolling tips (optional)
- Plastic rolling machine for cigarettes (optional)

Making a Filtered Joint by Hand

To roll a joint, first prepare your filter (inhibitor) if you want to reduce small pieces of MMJ getting in your mouth when you smoke.

Step 1: Tear off a sheet of rolling tips (I like the brand "Lefties"). From the short end of the paper, fold over about a half centimeter.

Step 2: Flip the paper over and fold over the other way and repeat until the entire paper is folded zigzag and looks like an accordion.

> ➢ You can roll a double filter (my preference because it makes the joint smaller – just right for a short smoke[x]); just do not tear the middle perforation on the sheet when you remove it from the pack. Fold the entire sheet from the short end in zigzag fashion.

Step 3: Now take a sheet of rolling paper (I like the "Zig-Zag" brand of slow burning 1-1/4" paper) and lay it down with the shiny adhesive side showing.

Step 4: Place your filter on the paper so that it will be covered by the paper (if you don't stick it well the filter will fall out of your joint), with the end of your filter flush with one end of your paper.

Step 5: Prepare your MMJ by picking it apart with your fingers or crushing it in a grinder. The smaller you grind your MMJ, the faster it will burn. You can find small hand-held manual grinders at your local smoke store or dispensary. Because too small a grind will burn your MMJ very quickly, I do not recommend grinding your bud in a coffee grinder unless you are preparing *medibles*.

Step 6: Fill your rolling paper with MMJ (or a tobacco/MMJ mix[y]) from the end of your filter to the end of the paper sheet.

---

[x] You will probably discover, like me, that it is challenging to stub out your joint without destroying it. That is why I prefer to make smaller joints that I can just smoke then toss.
[y] Mixing tobacco increases the strength of your MMJ, but you can also smoke straight MMJ in your joint. Because pipe tobacco is cut larger than cigarette tobacco, I have found cigarette tobacco easier to roll into my joints. A *joint* is pure weed rolled in a paper; a *spliff* is a mixture of weed and tobacco.

Step 7: Roll your filter and MMJ so that the shiny horizontal end of your paper remains visible.

Step 8: Carefully lick the shiny adhesive on the rolling paper and close your joint.

Your dispensary probably sells pre-rolled joints (usually without a filter), and you may wonder how they are able to roll the joints so cleanly and tightly. The company Raw makes a nifty and inexpensive plastic machine for rolling joints. I use the 79mm rolling machine (shown on left), which fits 1-1/4 rolling paper. You can find this on Amazon (http://www.amazon.com/RAW%C2%AE-Hemp-Plastic-Cigarette-Rolling-Machine/dp/B003ZNFTF0).

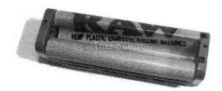

Rolling a joint in the machine takes a little practice, but after you get the hang of it this approach is phenomenally quicker and tighter than rolling by hand. Following are the steps for rolling a joint in the machine:

Rolling a Joint Using a Cigarette Machine

Step 1: Open the roller (with the movable side facing you) and place the desired amount of MMJ (or MMJ/tobacco mix) into it. Be sure it is spread evenly. If you want to insert a filter, place your pre-folded filter in the roller (to one end) first and then fill the rest of the roller with your MMJ.

Step 2: Close the roller.

Step 3: Using your thumbs over the top of the roller slowly roll towards you until you make one full rotation.

Step 4: Take your paper and place it into the closed opening of the roller. Make sure the sticky strip is at the top and is facing you.

Step 5: Using your thumbs on the front side of the roller, and your index fingers on the back side, slowly roll towards you until only the sticky strip is left in sight.

Step 6: Lick the sticky strip.

Step 7: Roll the stick strip in so it is no longer visible.

Step 8: Using your thumbs over the top of the roller, complete a few rotations to tighten and seal your joint.

Step 9: Open the roller and remove your joint.

Step 10: Smoke and repeat.

There are videos available on YouTube for "how to use a rolling machine for cigarettes."

Vaporizer

If you are not a cigarette smoker, you may find it challenging to smoke a joint until your lungs get used to it. My first smoking tool was a vaporizer, which has the benefit of letting you control the temperature so that you can release the THC without burning the carcinogens.

The potential harm caused by smoking MMJ can be minimized by using a vaporizer because vaporizers heat the active components in MMJ to a temperature below the ignition point of the cannabis. The vapors can be inhaled while combustion of plant material is avoided, thus preventing the formation of carcinogens such as poly-aromatic hydrocarbons, benzene, and carbon monoxide. In short, vaporizers give you a cooler and safer smoke.

The basic parts of a vaporizer are:

    A – vaporizer unit
    B – mouthpiece
    C – wand
    D – screen (a wire mesh filter inside the wand)
    E – plastic tubing
    F – temperature control and on/off knob
    G – heating element
    H – metal pick (not shown)

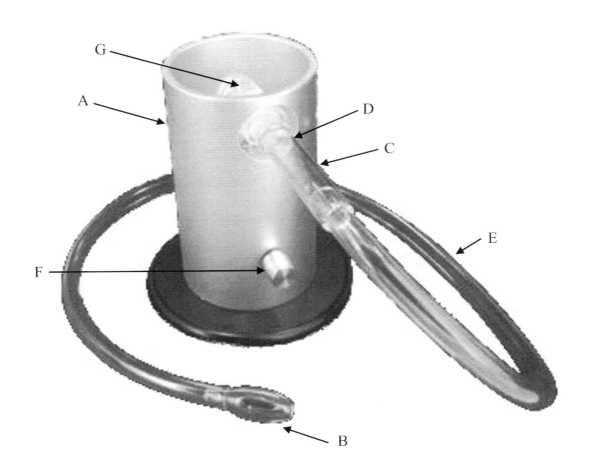

Using a Vaporizer

Step 1: Warm up your vaporizer by plugging it in and turning the heat dial about ¼ from all the way up. Your vaporizer may need 10-15 minutes to fully heat up.

Step 2: Prepare your MMJ by crushing or grinding it.

Step 3: Fill the wand loosely about half full with your MMJ. Do not pack your MMJ too tightly, as you need airflow around it to extract the THC.

Step 4: Place the open end of the wand (where your MMJ is) over your vaporizer's heating element.

Step 5: While holding the wand against the heating element, take the mouthpiece end of the tubing and inhale. Adjust the temperature of your vaporizer until you are able to produce white smoke when you exhale.

Step 6: To maximize each hit, remember to hold your breath as long as possible before exhaling.

Step 7: To get an even burn, stir and fluff up your MMJ with a metal pick[z] before each hit.

Step 8: When your MMJ has turned brown, it used up in your vaporizer.

Step 9: Using your metal pick, empty your used MMJ from your wand[aa] and refill.

---

[z] Usually sold with vaporizers, but any thin metal pick will do.
[aa] If you want to hold more MMJ, purchase a "fatty wand."

Until you get the hang of it, putting a new screen back in your wand can be frustrating. The benefits of having a fresh screen every few days, however, outweigh the chore of practicing a little until you can replace your screen quickly[bb]. Here are step-by-step instructions:

Replacing the Screen in Your Vaporizer Wand

Step 1: Remove the hose from your wand.

Step 2: Using a metal pick, remove the old screen by pushing it through your wand. The screen will bend to fit through the hole.

Step 3: Take your new screen (make sure it is the same size that you are replacing[cc]) and bend it into the shape of a shallow bowl.

Step 4: Using your pick, carefully push the screen into the mouthpiece end of your wand until it touches the lip of the hourglass.

Step 5: With your pick, flip the screen over inside the wand so that the screen is convex (like a bubble) on top of the hourglass. This is the part that takes a little practice ☺. If you flip your screen correctly, an edge of the screen will catch the inside lip of the hourglass.

Step 6: Push the screen into place with your pick.

[bb] If you are new to vaporizing, buy at least 10 screens so that you have enough to learn with. Your first replacement attempts will probably bend your screens, making them unusable.
[cc] The standard vaporizer wand screen size is 15mm, but it is always a good idea to bring an old screen with you when buying a new pack of screens at the smoke store.

Pipe

After a few years of experimentation, I personally have found a tobacco pipe to be the easiest and most cost-effective way to smoke MMJ. Although you are inhaling the burning MMJ (a lung cancer risk), the ease of use and the immediate, strong effect makes the tobacco pipe my MMJ tool of choice. I like vaporizing, but after a year I found that I needed to use it practically constantly in order to attain the same level of high as when I first started using MMJ. I spend much less money on MMJ using a pipe than when I vaporized (and prepared medibles).

Pipes come in many shapes, sizes, and materials including glass, wood, metal and stone. For our purposes, we will group MMJ pipes as either (a) water pipe, or (b) dry pipe.

There are three basic types of pipes that use water:

1. Water pipe
2. Bong
3. Hookah

Water pipe. A water pipe (shown on next page) lets the user slowly draw the smoke through a hose and water. Water pipes are small, almost hand-held; they are just like regular pipes but have water in them. A *bubbler*, for example would be a water pipe. A bubbler is a combination of a bong and a regular pipe. The bubbler has water in it to filter but it does not have a slide to pull out, only a *carb* (hole).

Parts of a Water Pipe

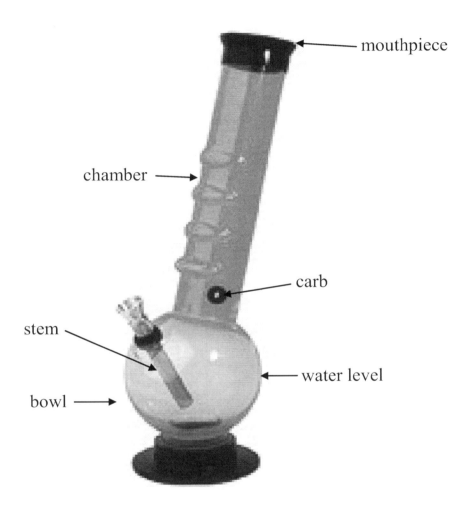

How to Smoke a Water Pipe

Step 1: Place your MMJ in the bowl. Fill your water pipe until the water level rises halfway up the stem.

Step 2: Cover the carb with your thumb and light the bowl.

Step 3: Pull air through the water pipe until you get a steady bubbling of smoke through the water.

Step 4: When your lungs start to hurt a little, let go of the carb and gently pull in the trapped smoke. If your lungs feel fine as you inhale, save a little lung space for the trapped smoke then let go of the carb and inhale.

Bong. A bong (shown below) is similar to a water pipe but the effect is different. When using a bong, the smoke passes the water very quickly and shoots right up into your lungs. Although the effect of a water pipe is more relaxed, you can feel the effect of a bong hit immediately. Because the bong chamber is much larger than a bowl, smoking a bong can be very effective.

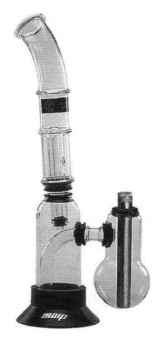

Bongs tend to be a larger than water pipes. They hold more water and more smoke, so you have to pull a little harder to get a lot of smoke up. Bongs and water pipes both have water, but bongs do not have a carb on them. Water pipes have a carb and a built-in bowl; bongs have a downstem and a slide or bowl.

A bong may be constructed from any air- and water-tight vessel by adding a bowl and stem apparatus (or *slide*) which guides air downward to below water level whence it bubbles upward (hence the name "bubbler") during use. To get fresh air into the bong and harvest the last remaining smoke, a hole known as the *carburetor, carb, choke, bink, rush* or *shotty*, somewhere on the lower part of the bong above water level, is first kept covered during the toke, then opened.

A bong can be many different styles but the basic design is universal. Smoke is pulled through water which gets rid of some carcinogens and makes for a much smoother hit.

The word *bong* is an adaptation of the Thai word *baung* which refers to a cylindrical wooden tube, pipe, or container cut from bamboo, and which also refers to the bong used for smoking. The word *bong* is said to be related to weed smoking. Since it is illegal to sell bongs *per se*, retailers call them "water pipes," which implies that the pipe will be used to smoke tobacco.[dd]

[dd] It has been said that the main difference between bongs and water pipes is that one is spelled B-O-N-G and the other one is legal.

How to Smoke a Bong[93]

Step 1: **Fill your bong with cold water.** Cold water will cool down the smoke so that more can be inhaled. Some users prefer filling their bong with ice, and then adding just enough cold water so that the bong makes a bubbling sound when inhaled through. Some users prefer very hot water because the steam helps bring moisture into the lungs.[ee]

Step 2: **Check your water level.** Make sure that the water level in your bong is not too high. The water level should be low enough so that it does not spill out the slider as you bend down to take a hit. The water level should also be deep enough to fully cleanse the smoke (at least 3" above the bottom of your slider). The more water that touches the surface of the smoke, the smoother.

Step 3: **Pack your bowl.** Make sure that your bowl is not so full that your MMJ will fall out of your bowl. Pack your MMJ to a medium-tight consistency. You want to get as much material in your bowl as possible while still being able to pull air through it with each inhale.

Step 4: **Place your mouth against the opening, forming a seal with your lips.** Make sure that the entire opening is covered or you will not be able to draw any smoke through your bong.

Step 5: **Grip the bong, holding one hand on the slider.** The slider is the stem of your bong which contains the bowl.

Step 6: **Hold a lighter up to your bowl[ff] while inhaling.** Your chamber should fill up with thick smoke.[gg] Inhale until you feel a sufficient amount of smoke has filled the chamber. When your lungs are about ¾ full, slide out the slider and inhale the remaining smoke from the chamber.

[ee] The drying effect of smoke, not the heat of the smoke, is the main reason people cough while using a water bong.
[ff] Not so close that you light your herb on fire.
[gg] Called the "milk."

Hookah. A hookah has a very large bowl and 2-4 hoses, having been designed to for multiple people to smoke it at the same time.[hh] Like a vaporizer, a hookah heats the tobacco more than it burns it.

Parts of a Hookah[94]

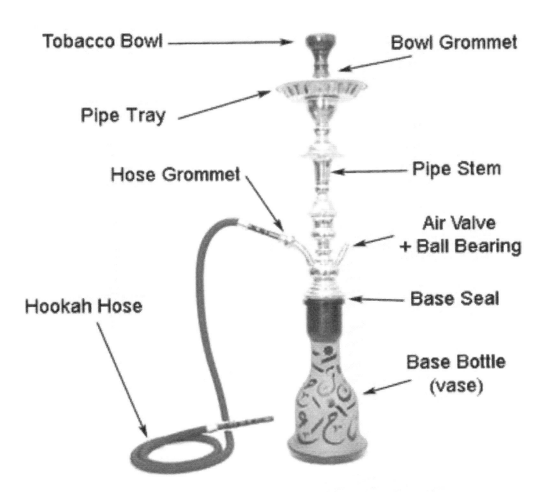

[hh] As opposed to a bong, which has a small bowl and only one person can smoke it at a time.

Base

The hookah base is typically made out of glass. It can be any variety of colors; usually the hookah base has an etched or painted design. They also come in a wide variety of shapes.

Pipe

The pipe is the body of the hookah and is typically made of brass, stainless steel, or tin. It has two important attachments that you need to know about. The hose socket is where you attach the hose to the pipe. The release valve is a one-way valve that is unscrewed to reveal the tiny small bearing inside it. If the smoke in your hookah becomes too strong, the release valve allows you to gently blow through the hose, which will force the smoke in the base out through the release valve. Be careful though, because if the valve is clogged and you blow forcefully on the hose it can force water up out of the pipe or blow the hot coals out of the bowl.

Hose

The hose is usually gaudy, brightly colored, and elaborately decorated. The hose is usually made of ribbed rubber, while the ends of the hose are made of wood. One end of the hookah hose fits into the pipe hose socket, while the other end has a handle and a small metal mouthpiece.

Bowl

The bowl is made of clay, and has five small holes. Rare bowls have only one large hole. The bowl holds the shisha tobacco and the coal.

Coal Tray

The coal tray is a convenient resting place for tongs and other items you may need while using your hookah. It also catches some ash that blows out from the coals.

Tongs

Tongs let you handle the hot coals without getting burnt.

Rubber/Plastic Collars

Used to ensure there is a tight seal at various connections between the hookah's parts. These are optional and are usually found on more expensive hookahs.

Wind Cover

The wind cover is a light, metal cylinder that rests on the coal tray and protects the bowl and its content from wind, careless people, etc. This is also optional, but it is very handy to have.

Disposable Mouth Pieces

These are mostly used at hookah bars and clubs, for sanitation reasons.

Shisha Tobacco

This is what you smoke in a hookah. Shisha is a mixture of tobacco, molasses, fruit and flavor extracts and provides a flavorful smoking experience.

Coals

The coals you use needs to be the 'self-lighting' smokeless kind. The coals are manufactured specifically for burning incense and smoking shisha. Do not use regular charcoal because you would risk carbon monoxide poisoning.

How to Smoke a Hookah

Hookahs are smoked much differently than a bong.

Step 1: Pack the molasses tobacco (*shisha*) into the bowl

Step 2: Cover the bowl with tin foil

Step 3: Poke some small holes in the tin foil

Step 4: Place a hot coal on top of the tin foil

Step 5: Take your mouthpiece and smoke.

Dry pipe. For those of you who prefer a more portable means for smoking your MMJ, the dry pipe offers a solution. The most common dry pipes are made of glass or wood, though you can find pipes made from clay, stone, metal, synthetics and more.[ii]

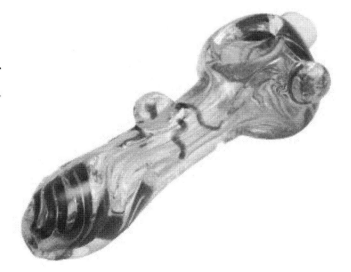

A glass pipe (on right) is popular for smoking MMJ, and works like a water pipe without the water.

[ii] Corncob pipes, literally made from the dried core of an ear of corn, are a part of Americana and are still in demand today.

How to Smoke a Glass Pipe

Step 1: Line your pipe bowl with a wire (or glass) mesh screen to prevent inhaling pieces of MMJ (optional).

Step 2: Place your MMJ in the pipe bowl. Do not pack too tightly, because you need airflow around the weed.

Step 3: Cover the side hole (*carb*) in your pipe with a finger or thumb.

Step 4: Light a flame (lighter or match) and hold it just above your bowl, without igniting your MMJ.

Step 5: Suck in through the pipe, pulling the flame into your MMJ.

Step 6: As you near the end of your inhalation, put out your flame, uncover the carb and release the rest of the smoke into your lungs.

Step 7: Hold your breath and long as you can, then exhale.

Step 8: Repeat.

 Glass pipes look cool and are visible part of marijuana culture. Glass pipes, however, are never mistaken for anything than what they are for. This makes glass pipes, in my opinion, impractical for use in public.
 Wooden pipes are fast and easy to use, and have the benefit of not standing out as drug paraphernalia. For this reason smoking MMJ with a wooden pipe has become my preference, plus the tobacco chamber on a wooden pipe is usually larger than the bowl on a glass pipe.

Parts of a Wooden Pipe

Pipe Stem

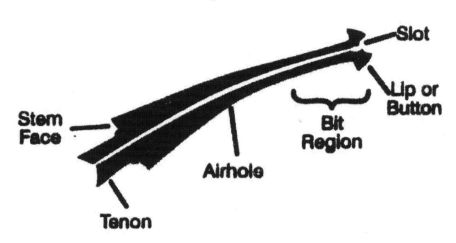

Pipe Bowl

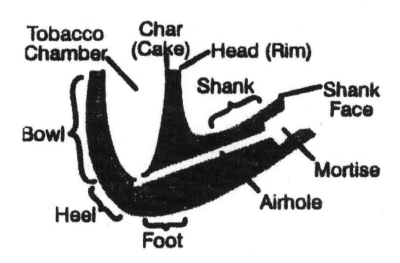

Illustrations courtesy of Stag Tobacconists, Colorado Springs, CO. Reprinted with permission.

How to Smoke a Wooden Pipe

You will need the following:

- Wooden pipe[jj]
- Pipe tobacco
- A few grams of crushed MMJ
- Wooden matches (my preference) or a butane lighter
- Ashtray
- Pipe cleaners
- Water or another beverage (optional)

Step 1: Fill the tobacco chamber (bowl) of your pipe by holding your pipe over your tobacco pouch (to catch loose tobacco) and sprinkling tobacco into the bowl. Once filled, tap the side of the pipe bowl with your knuckles[kk] to settle the tobacco. Add more tobacco and retap. Repeat until your tobacco chamber is full to the top with lightly packed tobacco.

[Steps 2-4 are optional:]

Step 2: Light your flame and hold it slightly above your bowl while taking light puffs through the mouthpiece. Your puffs should pull the flame into your tobacco. Expect to get an initial light (*char light*) each time you light a new bowl; this initial light will burn out.

Step 3: Puff on your pipe 5-6 times or so (do not inhale) while moving the flame around the entire bowl to get an even burn.

Step 4: Extinguish your pipe.[ll]

Step 5: Press a slight indentation in the tobacco in your bowl. You now have a ready tobacco base for your MMJ and/or hash.

[jj] Briar pipes are the most commonly sold pipes in stores.
[kk] Wooden pipes are soft and will dent if tap it on a hard surface.
[ll] I use my matchbook to put out my pipe after each hit I take, saving my tobacco and MMJ for future tokes throughout the day from a single bowl.

Step 6: Add your MMJ on top the tobacco in the chamber.

Step 7: Relight and smoke. Immediately extinguish your pipe while you hold your breath.

Step 8. Relight and smoke. After the MMJ has burned off, you can still use the tobacco base in your pipe and just add another pinch of MMJ (or hash) on top the ashes in your bowl. In order to delay *tongue bite*, I find it helpful to rap my pipe a few times to resettle/redistribute my leaf and then tamp the ashes down into the bowl (with my finger) before each smoke[mm]. You can probably get 2-5 strong tokes from one pipe bowl.

Step 9. When you have used up your tobacco base (you will get more of a bite when you smoke and/or you may experience harsh burning in your lungs), tamp out your tobacco chamber and start a new bowl.

Step 10. (optional) Tobacco pipe aficionados say to always smoke the whole bowl, in order to create an even cake layer in the tobacco chamber. I personally get too much bite after 2/3 of my tobacco is used, so I empty and fill with fresh tobacco (and MMJ).

> *If your pipe is not staying lit, you packed it too tightly. If you are burning your tongue or throat, you packed your pipe too loosely.*

As I alluded to earlier, one other advantage of using a tobacco pipe (versus a joint, vaporizer, or other type of pipe) is that it is easier to smoke in public without drawing attention to yourself. A friend of mine actually lit up a MMJ/tobacco mix in his briar pipe while standing next to a police officer without the officer giving my friend a second look.

[mm] This is opposite of when you use a vaporizer, where you want to fluff up your smoking mix before each toke.

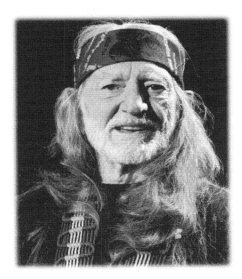

I think people need to be educated to the fact that marijuana is not a drug. Marijuana is a flower. God put it here....
— *Willie Nelson*

Chapter 5
Smoking Tips and Tricks[nn]

After two years of trial and error on my part to get the most effect out of my MMJ, I have compiled the following advice:

General Tips

1. **Do not forget to renew your MMJ id card before[oo] it expires!** Dispensaries are not permitted to sell MMJ to you with an expired card – the dispensary will not risk losing their business license in order to bend the rules, so do not ask them to. Each year before your card expires you need to see a MMJ-friendly physician again and get the paperwork completed and signed for your renewal.

[nn] If you have any additional advice to share, please e-mail us at tips@thetokebook.com so we can include your tip or trick in any future edition of this book. Thank you!

[oo] Prior to 2012, for example, Colorado law changed from allowing patients with expired cards (but proof of mailing in their renewal documentation) to still be able purchase MMJ from dispensaries. Now, all patients must show a valid card. With a wait of 30+ days for renewal processing, therefore, if you do not have your replacement MMID card in hand <u>before</u> your old card expires, you cannot legally buy MMJ.

2. To retain the freshness of your MMJ, store it in an airtight container (mason jars are popular) in a cool, dark, dry place. Some users store their MMJ in the refrigerator or freezer.

3. If you want to fill your lungs, remember to fully exhale (like you are blowing out the candles on your birthday cake) before you toke.

4. If you get too much of a high after smoking MMJ, do <u>not</u> put your head between your knees. This will cause blood to rush to your head and make your high even stronger.

5. Just like mixing medicines together, mixing MMJ strains can increase the effect. Try combining two or more strains of crushed MMJ in your joint, vaporizer, or pipe. Keep track of what you mixed, so you can create the combination again if you like it.

6. Dispensaries often do not label your purchase besides a warning label and the name of the strain. In order to keep track of which MMJ strains are helping you, I recommend you write the percent of Sativa/Indica on each container of MMJ you have.

7. THC is stored and absorbed in body fat, an important point to remember when calculating how MMJ (especially medibles) will affect you. People with a high BMI (body mass index) may feel the effects more, needing to consume less. For people with less body fat, adding fat with your consumption of cannabis will give a better effect. For example, eating nuts or avocados with your edible will help improve your absorption of THC.[95] I have also read that drinking milk increases THC absorption. Ginger and capcasin are both said to improve digestion and increase metabolism, thus they are used in preparing medibles. Lastly, supplementing with Vitamin C or potassium (drink some orange juice; eat a banana) helps absorb THC that is taken orally (medible or drinkable).

8. Regarding smoking, however, I have not discovered taking any particular supplement enhances the effect of MMJ. Generally, taking any medicine (including smoking MMJ) on an empty stomach increases its effect. Smoking on an empty stomach, I found, also can reduce the chance of nausea

9. Before rolling a joint, scrunch up the rolling paper to make it easier to work with.

10. Good quality pipe tobacco is best purchased at a pipe/cigar store, and is usually even less expensive (and much better quality) than pipe tobacco you can get at your local grocery store. I usually keep 100 grams of pipe tobacco in stock at home.

11. Mixing tobacco (cigarette or pipe) with your MMJ, I assure you, increases the effect of MMJ. It has been reported that tobacco increases THC absorption by 45%, a fact supported by my first-hand experience. I wrongly assumed that smoking straight MMJ was stronger, and that people who mixed it with tobacco were just doing it to economize on their MMJ. One evening, however, after smoking a joint before a concert I took a few puffs of my wife's cigarette. My head immediately went into the stratosphere (I also vomited up everything I had eaten earlier that day).[pp] So if there is one thing I do know, it is that smoking tobacco (even not mixed with MMJ, as was my first experience) definitely escalates MMJ's effects.

    Considering, then, that tobacco is three times less carcinogenic than MMJ,[qq] and mixing tobacco will make your MMJ stronger (and your bud last longer), why not smoke a combination of tobacco and MMJ?

    My MMJ doctor states that the anti-cancer effects of smoking MMJ cancel out the carcinogenic dangers of smoking it. Although I am not sure it has been medically proven (see p. 10), this would be nice if it were the case.

12. Which flavor pipe tobacco you smoke is a matter of personal preference. There are three main classes of pipe tobacco - Virginia, English and Aromatic.

    a) If you have smoked cigarettes you might like Virginia based tobaccos
    b) If you like big, bold flavors and smells you might like English style tobacco
    c) If you like some sweetness and a pleasant room aroma, Aromatics might be a good choice.

[pp] After my colossal trip came down, and my stomach settled, my pain relief from that combination of MMJ and tobacco helped make that one of the best concert experiences I had.
[qq] See p. 40

13. In a pinch, you can use cigarette tobacco in your pipe…but it tastes strong and burns quickly.

14. Your tobacco, like your MMJ, should have a degree of moisture to it when purchased. Be cautious about buying grocery store tobacco. Since grocery stores tend to not have much product turnover in their smokers' supplies, from my experience there is a good chance that the tobacco you buy at a grocery store might be stale and dry.

15. Though it may not always test so in a lab, I find that *bubble hash* is stronger than *sift (filtered) hash*.

16. Depending on your state laws, if you need to consume more than 2 oz. of MMJ per month your prescribing physician can issue you a *limits letter*. The limits letter will enable you to legally purchase a specific, larger amount per month based on your medical condition.

17. MMJ registry reciprocity currently only exists in Arizona, Delaware, Maine, Michigan, Montana and Rhode Island.[ᴨ] If you are flying to a state without reciprocity,

    ➢ Do not bring MMJ on an airplane
    ➢ Do not get caught mailing yourself your MMJ supply to your destination.

    The US Post Office and all US airports are under federal jurisdiction; MMJ is legal in certain states but not by the federal government.

18. Smoking can cause your nose to run. It is not a bad idea to have a handkerchief or tissues handy when you smoke.

19. To optimize your hit, try hyperventilating – exhale completely, inhale completely, then exhale completely again – before inhaling. Like a swimmer who maximizes the oxygen in his or her lungs before going underwater, hyperventilating will allow you to take a deeper, longer toke.

[ᴨ] See p. 13.

20. Try *stacking* your strains, smoking a different strain of MMJ (or hash) with each hit. You will need to have more than one joint, wand or pipe to do this effectively.

21. If you use a hand grinder for your weed, remember to periodically open the bottom chamber of your grinder where the dust (called *kief*) passes through the screen. Kief is high in THC content, so save it for smoking.

22. If you purchase a scale, an easy way to check its calibration is to put a nickel on the scale. A U.S. nickel weighs exactly 5 grams.

23. Is it dangerous to chew gum while smoking MMJ? Based on some (mostly anecdotal) information I found, some chemicals can adhere to the gum you chewing while smoking, possibly increasing the risk of developing cancer of the mouth or throat.

24. As you smoke, you may develop "smoker's cough,"[ss] as did I. Your family doctor can prescribe you an inhaler, which will help keep your cough at bay. My favorite inhaler is the Asmanex® Twisthaler®, which only needs to be used once a day. There are other inhalers, such as the Proair® HCA rescue inhaler, which you can use as needed. Just remember that the acids in inhalers can be damaging to your teeth, so brush your teeth immediately after using your inhaler (I use my inhaler once each evening, right before brushing my teeth).

25. If you have a stubborn cough that just does not want to clear from your lungs, try the following:

    ➢ Exhale completely then take a deep breath
    ➢ If that does not work, take another hit of your pipe and then try coughing again.

[ss] Stoners quip, "You don't get off until you cough."

26. Do you use a lighter for your pipe? Please review this important warning from Allan Bumgartner, chemist at CannLabs:

> The reader has probably seen lighters that are blackened on the plastic end from the practice of extinguishing a bowl of MMJ in a pipe after taking a hit. The molten plastic transferred to the MMJ in the bowl caused by this practice should be far more worrisome than properly extracted butane concentrates. The reason is that the transferred plastic is now smeared on the MMJ. The next hit from the pipe will be a combination of MMJ and molten plastic.
>
> The plastics that disposable lighters are made out of are usually Delrin plastic for Bic® brand lighters and PVC (polyvinyl chloride) plastic for less expensive brand lighters. According to the Material Safety Data Sheet (MSDS), when Delrin plastic is burned or combusted, carbon monoxide and formaldehyde gas are formed. Carbon monoxide is known to cause asphyxiation and formaldehyde gas is a known carcinogen. Consulting the other MSDS online, it states that when PVC plastic is burned, carbon monoxide and dioxin gas are formed. Carbon monoxide can asphyxiate and dioxin is a known carcinogen. It should generally be assumed that all burned plastics form carcinogens.
>
> It is recommended that the MMJ user use the metal end of a disposable lighter, rather than the plastic end, to extinguish the product in the bowl of a pipe. This eliminates the possibility of smoking melted plastic, containing carcinogens. Plus, the metal will not melt....To ensure that the medicine you are using remains as pure and unadulterated as when it was purchased, please use the metal end of your disposable lighter to extinguish the flame of your medicine between hits. Or, let the flame go out naturally. There is no reason to deliberately make your medicine harmful to you[96].

After reading Mr. Bumgartner's warning, I stopped using my lighter (see right) as a pipe extinguisher and now use a matchbook cover.

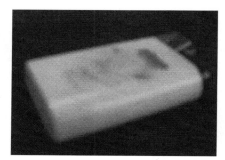

Bong Tips[97]

1. Very hot water will remove the most impurities, and very cold water will cool the smoke for a smoother hit. Be careful not to shatter your bong by changing water temperatures too extremely.

2. Use **fresh clean water** for smoking your product *every time* you smoke with your bong. Re-using dirty water defeats the purpose of your water as a filter in your bong.

3. If you feel a cough coming, pull your mouth away from the bong. Coughing into the bong with the slide still in will send the slide (and your smoking mix) flying out.

4. If you find your lungs have been destroyed from a toke and you are in pain, *take a few deep breaths* (although very painful) and it will take away the pain and ease after a few moments. Refreshing your lungs is one key to avoiding coughs and pain.

5. Leaving unchanged and rancid water can generate quite an unpleasant odor if left for long periods of time. To keep your bong nice-tasting and smooth, clean it with a simple mix of kosher (coarse) salt and rubbing alcohol. A few shakes and a soak will dissolve the black resin.

6. If you do cough and you find yourself feeling like you just sucked on the wrong end of a flame thrower, after you get fresh air into your lungs if your throat is still burning, usually drinking something sugary and non-carbonated (like Gatorade®) will help.

7. Pressing your lighter flat onto the slide (making it airtight) will help you pull the remaining bits of your mix.

8. Use your metal pick to stir up the remaining clogged up bits of product and ash from the slide after use, making it easier and smoother for the next person.

9. Instead of water, try using Gatorade® or some kind of light fruit juice (apple, white grape) in your bong.

10. Always pass the lighter with the bong to the next person to be sure to keep track of it.

11. To prevent bong water from splashing into your mouth, you can insert a *splash guard* (a barrier in the tube) after the percolators and before the ice catcher.

12. Daisy (or honeycomb) style glass pipe screens are available for bongs. Screens prevent your MMJ from being pulled through the hole, plus there is no metallic taste from a glass screen, though you can use a disposable metal screen in your bong.

    i. To use, place your screen over your bowl and pack your MMJ on top
    ii. Clean your glass screen with rubbing alcohol just like your bong.

13. To clean your bong, use rubbing alcohol and coarse salt. Shake around and dump in the toilet,[tt] then make sure to rinse out all salt and alcohol (with warm soapy water) before filling to smoke again.

14. When cleaning any glass products (bong, wand, mouthpiece, etc.), remember to completely wash out the alcohol with hot, soapy water so you are not smoking any alcohol residue.

[tt] Make sure you flush immediately or resin will stick to the side of your toilet bowl.

Vaporizer Tips

1. Warning: Do not use tobacco in your vaporizer. I tried a MMJ/tobacco mix in my vaporizer and all I got was a nasty tobacco taste. In short, just use only MMJ (weed or hash) in your vaporizer.

2. Do you want a quick way to fill your wand? Put your mouth to the mouthpiece and suck up your MMJ into your wand.

3. Replace your screen frequently (every few days or less). Replacement screens cost about 10 cents each (at your local smoke store or on-line), and you will immediately notice the ease of inhaling with a new screen in your wand.

4. Vaporizers do not work so well outdoors. In my experience, the ambient temperature and wind prevent the vaporizer element from getting hot enough. I use my vaporizer indoors and sit near a cracked window so I can exhale my smoke outside.

5. The speed at which you draw (inhale) from your vaporizer has a strong effect on how the MMJ in your wand burns. The slower you inhale, the hotter your MMJ will get (and the greater possibility of burning it). In order to get a good vapor (not smoke), you will want to experiment drawing slowly. If your vaporizer element is hot, inhale more quickly (to cool the air going through your wand).

6. Cleaning your wand and mouthpiece can be done easily with kosher salt and rubbing alcohol. When your wand is too dirty to see through, disconnect it (and your mouthpiece) from the plastic tubing. Remove the screen from your wand and throw it away. Place your wand and mouthpiece in a zip-lock freezer bag then fill with about ¼ cup of kosher salt and 1 cup of rubbing (isopropyl) alcohol. Seal the bag closed and swish it around to mix. Place the bag in your sink (in case of leaks), making sure that the wand and mouthpiece are covered with your alcohol/salt mixture.

   Within an hour (you can leave them soaking overnight if you want), your wand and mouthpiece will be as clean as new. Dump your bag out in the sink or toilet; rinse your wand and mouthpiece with warm soapy water; then dry with a paper towel (remember to dry inside your wand also). Insert a new screen into your wand (see p.54) and reconnect your wand and mouthpiece to your tubing.

7. Rather than clean your plastic tubing when it becomes dirty, you can smoke the inside residue. When your tubing has become a dark golden color, pull off your wand and mouthpiece, then cut the tubing lengthwise with a pair of scissors and scrape off the inside residue with the blade of your scissors or a butter knife. This residue is *very* smokeable with a high concentration of THC. Add the residue on top your MMJ the next time you vaporize.

8. I like to start my vaporizer at a low heat (about halfway to full power) and then gradually increase the temperature with each hit until I find the "sweet spot" on my vaporizer temperature knob. Continue increasing the temperature a little bit with each hit you take until your herb is used up, and you will maximize your MMJ.

9. If your screen is clogged (even after blowing from the vaporizer end of your wand to clear it) and you do not have a fresh screen handy, in a bind you can use a lighter to burn the residue off your old screen. Leave the screen in your wand, however, since the screen will probably get too bent if you remove it and try to put it back in your wand.

10. A portable vaporizer (shown on right) is something you might try. It at least gives you the flexibility to vaporize anywhere (the unit is small enough to fit in your pocket). Portable vaporizers use butane to heat your MMJ in a small bowl. My experience with portable vaporizers is that mine did not heat up enough[uu]. Besides, using a portable vaporizer in public is a lot more conspicuous than smoking a briar pipe (or even a joint).

11. If you do not have a metal pick, an unbent paperclip works as well.

[uu] New portable vaporizers continue to hit the market, and reports are that some of them heat up better.

Pipe Smoking Tips

1. You can clean your glass pipe the same way you clean the vaporizer wand – soak it in a solution of rubbing alcohol and salt.

2. When filling your tobacco pipe, pack the tobacco loosely (but tapped down) on the bottom. A smoking pipe is like a furnace which feeds the flame from the bottom. Packing your pipe too tightly on the bottom will make it difficult to draw air through the stem.

3. When holding onto your pipe between tokes, or storing your pipe for later, keep the pipe stem upright (they even make pipe stands for this). If you lay your pipe down, you might get a bitter drip of nicotine the next time you put your pipe in your mouth.

4. If you want a really strong hit, put a little bubble hash on top your pipe tobacco. For my pre-bedtime smoke, I place a piece of bubble hash on top my tobacco base, and then I add a layer of Indica MMJ on top. This will get you where you need to go![vv] ☺

5. Store your unused pipe tobacco like you do your MMJ – in an airtight container to keep from drying out.

6. Inhaling through a pipe sends hot air into your lungs (especially the longer you pull on your pipe). To control how much heat you are breathing in, relax your mouth around the mouthpiece and let some fresh air in. Inhaling you can also take puffs, taking in a little air between each puff.

7. If your pipe is clogged and you do not want to dump out a new bowl, cup the pipe bowl with the palm of your hand and lightly blow through the pipe slot a few times. There is a good chance you can get your pipe opened up again without wasting your tobacco/MMJ.

8. When you are ready to empty your bowl, you will find that a matchstick is ideal for prying out the used tobacco/MMJ. After you dump the bulk of the material,

---

[vv] I am often reminded of the Tom Petty song lyrics, ""Last dance with Mary Jane, One more time to kill the pain…"

empty your bowl completely by lightly tapping into your palm and then blowing a few puffs through your pipe before refilling it with fresh tobacco/MMJ.

9. A good cake insulates the bowl and allows good air flow around the tobacco which promotes a clean, even burn and helps keep the tobacco lit. A good cake also prevents bowl burn outs and keeps your pipe burning cool and dry. The ideal cake is about the thickness of a dime or a nickel (US). Serious pipe smokers will regularly trim the cake to a thin even level inside their tobacco chamber; the tool used for this is called a *pipe reamer*. I just use a butter knife to trim the cake in my pipe once a month or so, though I'm sure a pipe reamer is probably more effective.

10. Here are some fun smoking tricks you can learn:[ww]

    ➢ French inhale – After taking a hit, open your mouth (letting the smoke flow out slowly). Then lightly inhale that smoke through your nose. If done right, the smoke will gradually flow out of your mouth and directly into your nose. You can then draw the rest of the smoke into your mouth or continue to inhale through your nose until the hit is completely finished.

    ➢ Snap inhale – After taking a hit, while the smoke is still in your mouth, curl your tongue upwards toward the roof of your mouth. Next, open your lips a bit and snap your tongue down. Finally, let the smoke float out of your mouth for a moment before you quickly inhale.

    ➢ Smoke rings – Take a hit and let your mouth fill with smoke (before or after you inhale). Form your lips into the shape of an "O" then quickly expel some of the smoke out of your mouth with the back of your tongue as you exhale. A tiny puff of smoke should emerge in the shape of a ring. You can change the size of the ring you exhale by varying the amount of space between your lips. Also, you can flex your throat muscles rapidly and shoot out rings in rapid-fire bursts. With enough practice, you may be able to shoot out a large ring and then quickly send a smaller ring speeding through the center of the large ring.

[ww] The smoking tricks above were generously contributed by Bud S. Moker, Th.C. at http://smokingwithstyle.com

11. Below are photos of two briar pipes. The shape does make a difference. I used the top shape (straight pipe) for over a year until the stem wore out. The bottom (bent) pipe is the shape like I have now (my favorite pipe brand is Peterson® of Dublin), and I definitely can tell that it smokes cooler than the straight pipe. A cooler smoke is easier on the lungs, so I recommend a curved pipe if you can find one in your price range. An inexpensive straight pipe can be found for less than $40, and decent curved pipes start around $90.

Straight Pipe

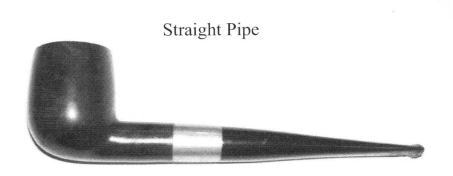

Curved Pipe

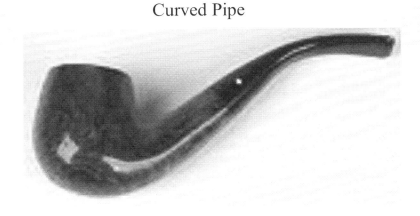

12. Instead of a slot at the end of the mouthpiece, some pipes have an air hole on the top of the mouthpiece. With this pipe design the smoke hits your palate first, which provides a more pleasant taste experience. You also do not get as many small tobacco pieces (if any) in your mouth or throat when you inhale – just remember to keep your pipe pointed downward so the slot is against your palate, not pointing down your throat. Highly recommended.

13. If you do not want to breathe in the butane from your lighter, use wooden matches[xx] (my preference). I still keep a lighter with me when I am out, however, in case it is too windy outdoors to get a match lit. After learning about the chemicals released when using a plastic lighter to extinguish my pipe (see pp. 73-74), I now also carry an old matchbook for extinguishing my pipe.

14. If you clean your pipe too frequently, you will wear out the stem from taking your pipe apart. You <u>do</u> want to clean your pipe regularly, however, because the build-up in the mouthpiece worsens the taste of your smoke.

15. In my previous edition of *The Toke Book* I wrote, "I clean my pipe every other day or so, depending on how much I have smoked." Since then, I have begun cleaning my pipe after every bowl. For a cleaner smoke and a better taste, I now highly recommended thoroughly cleaning your pipe with a pipe cleaner (at least after each bowl).

16. If you run your pipe cleaner through your pipe stem and it is covered in black, it is definitely time to clean your pipe. If you run your pipe cleaner through your pipe stem and it is only a light brown on the end of the pipe cleaner, you are probably cleaning your pipe too often.

17. If your throat burns when inhaling through your pipe (and your tobacco is not packed too loosely), you may be pulling too hard. With a pipe, you do not need to as draw nearly as hard as you would on a bong or vaporizer. Try pulling on your pipe gently (it does not take much to keep your pipe lit) and you will probably get a cooler smoke and less throat burn (*tongue bite*). You can also try packing down your tobacco/MMJ a little tighter in your bowl.

[xx] Paper matches burn fast, which can be a problem if you are moving the flame around your bowl to get an even burn. I personally use heavy kitchen matches.

18. If you get a nasty bitter taste when you put your pipe stem in your mouth, it is time to clean your pipe.

19. Experiment with your pipe bite. Rather than biting your pipe stem right at the lip (button), try taking a little more stem in your mouth (1/2") and you should find that your throat opens more and you get a deeper toke.

20. To get an optimal toke, fully seal your lips around the stem while inhaling. You will probably still need to let a little air in through the corners of your mouth, or puff your pipe. In general, a full seal on your stem help you will maximize the amount of MMJ into your lungs.

21. If you can afford it, avoid using the tobacco powder that is left in your bag after you smoke the tobacco leaf. Powder and very small bits of tobacco are more likely to clog your pipe – or worse, get sucked through the pipe into your throat when you smoke.

22. If you hate getting bits of tobacco in your mouth (like I do), after you pack your pipe chamber (but before lighting your pipe), suck through your mouthpiece, catching the tobacco bits on your tongue. Spit out, light your pipe and smoke.

23. To clean your pipe, separate the stem from the bowl and clean both with a thin pipe cleaner (see following page).

24. Do not clean your wooden pipe with water. The pipe will soak up water and your pipe will eventually crack when you smoke it.

25. Tapered pipe cleaners (my favorite brand is Bryco®) are ideal – the smaller end fits into your stem slot, and the thick end is great for cleaning your pipe bowl.

26. For a quick pipe cleaning, especially if you have no pipe cleaners handy:

    1. Empty your bowl
    2. Separate your pipe and stem
    3. Blow firmly through the slot in the stem
    4. Blow firmly through the pipe bowl (the mortise end, not the tobacco chamber end)
    5. Reassemble your pipe, fill, and smoke.

27. Stores sell varieties of fuzzy- and bristle-type pipe cleaners with different thicknesses, some of which may be too thick for your specific pipe. Make sure what you purchase will fit into your pipe stem.

Cleaning Your Tobacco Pipe

1. Separate the stem from the bowl and wipe down the tenon and shank face.

2. Set down the bowl for cleaning later.

3. Pass a new pipe cleaner through the stem. If your pipe has a mouthpiece slot, try feeding the pipe cleaner in through the tenon out the slot. If your pipe has a mouthpiece air hole, you will find it easier to feed your pipe cleaner in through the air hole and out through the tenon.

4. Bend the same pipe cleaner, set down the stem and pick up the bowl.

5. Run the doubled-over pipe cleaner through the mortise to the tobacco chamber a couple of times. If your mortise is narrow, you may only be able to run the unbent pipe cleaner through.

6. Use the doubled-over pipe cleaner to swab out the tobacco chamber.

7. IMPORTANT: Blow strongly through your pipe bowl (from the mortise end) in order to clear out any debris leftover from cleaning your pipe.

8. Reconnect the stem and bowl. Tap the bowl (I do it in the palm of my hand) to remove any loose cake. Blow out anything left inside, and your pipe is ready to refill.

9. Once a week or so, I take a used matchstick and scrape out the inside of my tobacco chamber to remove excess cake build-up. Once every few months, I use a butter knife to scrape out excess cake build-up inside my bowl.

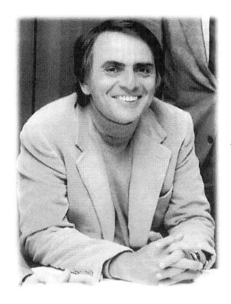

The illegality of cannabis is outrageous, an impediment to full utilization of a drug which helps produce the serenity and insight, sensitivity and fellowship so desperately needed in this increasingly mad and dangerous world.

– Carl Sagan

Chapter 6
Conclusion

If this book has helped you, then I have accomplished my goal. I hope that you have been able to use this manual to navigate the various ways to enjoy MMJ. As a fibromyalgia sufferer, I also hope that you have acquired an increased understanding of chronic pain and stress, and that you will encourage those around you to be more tolerant of people with invisible disabilities and their need to use MMJ.

As the song "Walking on the Sun" by Smash Mouth goes, "It ain't no joke I'd like to buy the world a toke and teach the world to sing in perfect harmony …" Good luck with your MMJ smoking; I hope it gives you relief!

If you have any good ideas to share about smoking MMJ, please contact me at jeff@thetokebook.com. The legal landscaping is rapidly changing for the good of pain management. Let's keep spreading the word. In the process of educating those who can get relief through MMJ we will also help remove society's stigma against weed smoking.

Glossary of Key Terms

Ace - Type of joint sold at medical marijuana dispensaries and clinics.

Antiemetic – A drug that is effective against vomiting and nausea. Over the counter (OTC) medicines that help against vomiting are Kaopectate, Pepto-Bismol. Dramamine is an OTC medicine that helps against nausea.

BC Bud - A particularly high-grade marijuana which from British Columbia.

Black Ganga - Marijuana resin oil sold at only some medical marijuana dispensaries and clinics.

Black Hash - Strong hashish usually associated with black resin. Currently hashish is allowed in most permissive marijuana states.

Blunt – a cigar stuffed with marijuana.

Bomber - Slang term used to describe a fat marijuana cigarette.

Bong - A large water pipe with a detachable bowl used for smoking medicinal marijuana. Smoking with a bong or vaporizer is supposedly healthier for the lungs since it is cooler air being breathed. There are two basic types of bongs – (a) grommet, and (b) glass on glass (GonG). A grommet bong uses a rubber ring that is placed on the bowl's stem to create an air tight seal with the down stem. Grommets are usually found on acrylic or ceramic bongs. A GonG bong uses a glass joint that is flush with the bowl to create an air tight seal between bowl and bong. GonG bongs are almost always better quality then grommet bongs, and thus more expensive.

Boron - A trace fertilizer necessary for the healthy growth of organic marijuana plants.

Bowl - A unit of measurement relating to one marijuana serving from a pipe.

Brick - Roughly one kilogram of marijuana.

Bubbler - A smaller handheld water pipe with a bowl used for smoking medicinal marijuana

Cannabinoids – A class of chemicals compounds and elements found in cannabis that includes the active ingredients in marijuana. There are currently three classes of cannabinoids:

1. Phytocannabinoids occur in plants, such as marijuana
2. Endocannabinoids occur naturally in the brain
3. Synthetic cannabinoids are created in laboratories and are not known to exist naturally

The three most discussed cannabinoids in the medical marijuana debate are (i) delta-9-tetrahydrocannabinol (delta 9-THC); (ii) cannabidiol (CBD); and (iii) cannabinol (CBN):

THC (Tetrahydrocannabinol) gets a user high. A larger proportion of THC will produce a stronger high. Without THC you don't get high. THC is responsible for most of the cerebral (mental) effects of cannabis. Besides potentially inducing feelings of euphoria and happiness, THC can cause people to feel anxious, nervous, or paranoid.

CBD (Cannabidiol) increases some of the effects of THC and decreases other effects of THC. Larger amounts of CBD tend to relax both mind and body, and decrease feelings like anxiety, nervousness, and paranoia. Cannabis that has a high level of THC and low level of CBD will produce a very strong cerebral high. The body may feel more physically energetic when compared to ingesting cannabis with larger levels of CBD.

Cannabis that has a high level of both THC and CBD will produce a strong cerebral high. The body will feel somewhat relaxed and heavy. At lower dose sizes, physical activity is possible (with effort). As the dose size increases, the body will feel more relaxed and heavy. This makes physical activity require more effort. Fresh hashish is an example of a cannabis product with high levels of both THC and CBD.

Cannabis that has low levels of THC and high levels of CBD will produce more of a stoned feeling. The mind feels relaxed and dull, the body feels relaxed and heavy, and there is a decreased interest in engaging in physical activity.

CBN (Cannabinol) is produced as THC ages. High levels of CBN tend to make a person feel messed up rather than high. CBN levels can be kept to a minimum by storing cannabis products in a dark, cool, airtight environment.

Cannabis - Also known as marijuana, weed, hemp, pot, ganja, reefer, and a hundred other slang descriptions, many of which are contained in this glossary.

Cannabis Club – An organized group of patients and/or caregivers joining together to supply cannabis to patients. Although some cannabis clubs are said to be well-run and work closely with local and state governments, it continues to be a <u>federal</u> crime to have or use marijuana for any purpose. In October 2001 and February 2002, the DEA raided and closed several cannabis clubs in California. In the process, the DEA confiscated medical records and arrested some participants. Many individuals were charged with crimes relating to those operations.

Cannabis Indica - One of two principle strains of the marijuana plants – indica and sativa. Each has their own unique effect. See *Indica*.

Cannabis Sativa - Known as the opposite strain to indica, it is one of two major strains of the marijuana plant – indica and sativa. Each has their own effect. See *Sativa*.

Carb - The hole found on pipes and bongs. A thumb is placed over it while taking a hit and released just before the user is done inhaling, clearing the smoke from the chamber of the device.

Carcinogenic – A substance or agent producing or inciting cancer.

Caregiver – A person who has agreed to undertake responsibility for managing the health and well-being of a person. In some states, a patient's Primary Caregiver is afforded the same protections from arrest and sanctions as the medical marijuana patient they care for.

CB1 / CB2 Receptors - Cannabis-based molecules found on the surfaces of brain cells, that enable these cells to communicate with neurotransmitters, hormones, and other messenger molecules.

Cake – The burned residue that builds up inside the bowl of a pipe. Also called *char*.

Caviar – Cannabis caviar is an expensive (but powerful!) treatment of MMJ bud that is starting to become available at dispensaries in California and Colorado. Caviar is made by soaking top-shelf marijuana buds in strong (30-80% THC) hash oil. After the hash oil is soaked into the bud, the now *infused* bud is then rolled in kief and slightly baked in order to dry.

Char Light - The first time tobacco/MMJ catches the flame when first lighting a pipe. The char light will burn out.

Chronic - A term used to describe a particularly potent form of marijuana that is popular in most medical marijuana dispensaries.

Cigarette (rolling) paper – Thin strips of paper with a lickable adhesive on one side; for rolling joints.

Clone - A branch clipping taken from a larger "mother" plant. With the correct care, the main branches of the plant can be rooted and used to start a new plant with the exact genetic makeup of the original plant. This is a well-known technique used by experienced marijuana cultivators to grow new plants without the use of seeds, so that they can keep their entire crop feminized and keep the flowers seed-free. Additionally, the use of clones allows for a grower to skip the early plant cycles and generally produce flowering buds quicker than starting growth from seeds.

Cobalt - A type of fertilizer used for growing organic medical marijuana.

Controlled Substance - A drug or other substance, or immediate precursor, included in schedule I, II, III, IV, or V of the U.S. Government's Controlled Substances Act.

Couchlock - When you get a very strong body high and cannot get up off the couch; usually obtained when smoking Indica weed.

DEA - The United States Drug Enforcement Administration, whose main purpose is to enforce the controlled substances laws and regulations of the United States.

Decriminalization - To remove or reduce the criminal classification or status of, or repeal a strict ban on while keeping under some form of regulation. This term is used in regards to medical marijuana to refer to a lessening of the laws for possession or use of marijuana.

Dispensary - Usually referring to a state approved medical marijuana outlet in which medical marijuana is legally sold. A patient's access to a medical marijuana dispensary requires a medical marijuana identification card (also known as an MMID card or "medically approved marijuana prescription").

Drug - A substance used as a medication or in the preparation of medication.

Drug Abuse - Use of a drug either without prescription or in excess of the recommended or prescribed dosage.

Drug Diversion - Giving or selling a drug lawfully obtained to another who has not the permission to use or obtain that drug.

Drug Reform - A change in the drug laws, most usually referred to in terms of lessening the laws for use or possession of a drug.

Ear Wax – Named so for its yellow waxy appearance, ear wax is a condensed form of marijuana extract, like hashish but not as hard, which can be smoked.

Enhanced bud - Marijuana buds that have been soaked in hash oil and/or rolled in kief.

Flowering - The act of major and expansive flowering of the cannabis plant.

Flushing – The process of rinsing marijuana plants (and soil) of excess, and potentially dangerous, salts and chemical nutrients.

Gateway Theory - The theory that experimenting with one drug will naturally lead the person to try other, more harmful drugs.

Genus - A category of biological classification ranking between the family and the species. Cannabis, for example, is a genus in flowering plant family.

Ghee - Liquid butter containing extracted THC; used for baking and preparing medibles.

Glandular Trichomes - Microscopic features used to identify herbal cannabis or cannabis resin. They produce an exudate containing cannabinoids and are located mostly around the flowering tops of female plants of *Cannabis sativa*.

Gram - The legal weight unit usually describing a small amount of medical marijuana or medically prescribed hashish.

Grass – One of the most common terms referring to smokeable marijuana.

Grinder – A manual appliance for chopping MMJ into small pieces, such as for making a joint.

Hashish (Hash) - The unadulterated resin from the flowering tops of the female hemp plant (*cannabis sativa*). Hashish is made from removing the trichomes from female cannabis plants and compressing them into small blocks than can be smoked, chewed, or swallowed in a liquid. Common forms of hash sold by dispensaries are *bubble* or *sift*, named by the process used to make it.

Hash Oil - A dark green or black tar-like material made by solvent extraction of either cannabis resin or herbal cannabis. Hash oil may contain up to 30-50% THC.

Hemp - A soft, durable fiber produced from the Cannabis plant. Hemp is one of the earliest domesticated plants and has a variety of uses. It is also very environmentally friendly. Typically Cannabis Sativa is used for hemp, while Cannabis Indica is not strong enough and is used for psychoactive or medical uses. Hemp contains less than 0.3% THC, which has no effect on the body. Hemp can be used to make paper, fabric, plastic, building materials, and biofuels, and can also be used by farmers as weed control and water filtration. The hemp seed is high in protein as well as beneficial omega fatty acids when eaten and has a variety of culinary uses. Hemp products are sometimes sold at dispensaries.

Hermaphrodite - A self-seeding marijuana plant including male and female flowers.

High Intensity Light - A type of light, more energy efficient than fluorescent lamps for purposes of growing marijuana.

Hit – A single inhalation and exhalation of MMJ, from any means (joint, vaporizer, pipe). Also called a "toke."

Honey Blunt – A marijuana cigar sealed with honey.

Hookah - A Middle Eastern smoking water pipe that can accommodate multiple smokers at one time. These are sold in many medical dispensaries and smoke shops.

Hybrid - The resultant offspring from marijuana plants of different breeds.

Indica - Indica marijuana is recognized by its compact growing style with short broad leaves and dark green color. Usually growing between 3 and 6 feet tall, mature indica plants emit a strong skunky smelling aroma. The smoke produced by these types of marijuana is generally thick and dense and considered by some to be on the harsh side. The medicinal results from indica dominant strains are most often described as more of a "body effect". Chronic pain sufferers will often find the most relief from 100% indica strains because of the extremely potent levels of THC that provide a natural pain reliever. Indicas are also helpful in treating stress and anxiety symptoms by providing an overall sense of relaxation and sedation similar to many anti-anxiety prescription medications.

IND Program - The Investigational New Drug (IND) Program is a program sponsored by the FDA which allows researchers to test new drugs prior to approval.

Infused Flower – MMJ bud that has been soaked in hash oil in order to increase its potency.

Infusion – Soaking MMJ bud in a liquid (usually hash oil) in order to transfer the THC from the liquid into the bud.

Initiatives - A procedure enabling a specified number of voters by petition to propose a law and secure its submission to the electorate or legislature for approval.

Inline Ash Catcher - An ash catcher usually built into the bong. An ash catcher acts as a second chamber that filters and cools the smoke before it enters the bong.

IOM Report - The 1999 report by the Institute of Medicine that examined the medical use of marijuana.

Joint - A cannabis cigarette; also referred to as a doobie, reefer or spliff.

Kief (or Keef) – The fine powder collected from marijuana, usually from a grinder or pollen press or left at the bottom of a bag, consisting of crystals (trichomes), bud hairs, and small particles of plant material. Good quality kief always has a much higher THC (the main cannabinoid) content than marijuana bud itself. It tends to therefore induce stronger highs when smoked than marijuana.

Lid - Slang for roughly one ounce of marijuana.

Limits letter – Legal authorization from your primary caregiver that because of your medical condition, you require purchasing more than the state limit (usually 2oz.) of MMJ per month.

Marijuana - Dried leaves and flowers of the plant Cannabis sativa L., used for the variety of psychoactive and physiological effects it has when ingested. Marijuana can be vaporized, eaten, or smoked. The word *marijuana* is a Mexican term that originally was applied to low-quality tobacco; the name also could have come from Mariguana, the name of one of the Bahamian islands. Some common street names for marijuana are: weed, pot, grass, herb, ganja, nugget, buddha, mary jane, pottery, herbal refreshment, bud, chronic, and left-handed tobacco.

Marijuana Plant - Usually referring to the male species of the cannabis plant.

Marijuana Lawyers - A collection of lawyers who are committed to the legal rights of the accused in criminal cases involving the illegal use of marijuana, as well as providing legal advice for lawfully operating medical marijuana dispensaries and clinics.

Medical Marijuana (MMJ) - The term used to describe organically grown marijuana in states that have legalized the medicinal use of marijuana.

Medical Marijuana Card - Also known as MJ Cards and Medical Pot ID Cards. It refers to the highly regulated state programs in about thirteen states that legally permit the use of medical marijuana for medicinal purposes. The marijuana card is usually issued by the recommending medical doctor along with a confidential patient identification number that later becomes part of a protected and anonymous database that can be accessed by law enforcement.

Medical Necessity - The common law legal doctrine that an illegal action to prevent a greater harm is not a crime, i.e. if an individual steals a boat to rescue a drowning person, the stealing of the boat is not considered a crime.

Medicine - A substance or preparation used in treating disease; something that affects well-being.

Milk – The thick, white smoke that fills a bong before it is inhaled.

Medibles - Foods (i.e., brownies, cookies, chocolates) or drinks (carbonated and noncarbonated) prepared with extracted THC. Medibles are absorbed in the stomach as opposed to smoking MMJ into the lungs.

Mortise – Part of a pipe bowl, where the stem connects to the shank face of the bowl

Narcotic - A drug that in moderate doses dulls the senses, relieves pain, and induces profound sleep but in excessive doses causes stupor, coma or convulsions.

NIDA - The National Institute on Drug Abuse is a U.S. government agency whose primary mission is "to lead the Nation in bringing the power of science to bear on drug abuse and addiction." NIDA is currently the only agency in the U.S. contracted to supply marijuana for research and IND programs.

NORML - The National Organization for the Reform of Marijuana Laws. A nonprofit organization focused on promoting the legal rights of marijuana smokers.

Nostrum - A medicine of secret composition recommended by its preparer but usually without scientific proof of its effectiveness.

Oil - Also known as concentrates, it is the high THC resin oil from different types of hashish or marijuana.

Paraquat - An herbicide (weed killer) once promoted by the United States for use in Mexico to destroy marijuana plants. After research found that this herbicide was dangerous both to workers who applied it to the plants and to people who smoked the marijuana harvested from them, Paraquat was banned in the United States, although it is still legal for some uses in Mexico.

Percolator - A filtering and cooling chamber that sits in the bong's tube. There are a few kinds of percolators, the most common ones being *tree percolators* and *dome percolators*.

Physician Recommendation - In medical marijuana, since a "prescription" for marijuana is not permitted under U.S. law, many MD's will recommend or approve marijuana for medical use, feeling this action is protected under the U.S. Constitution's 1st Amendment right to free speech.

Pipe - A tube of wood, clay, hard rubber, blown glass or other material, with a small bowl at one end, used for smoking tobacco or marijuana

Pipe Reamer – A metal device used to scrape off (or trim) cake residue in a wooden pipe tobacco chamber.

Pull – To inhale from a joint, vaporizer or pipe.

Pot - Slang for marijuana/cannabis. The word is rooted in the Mexican Spanish "potiguaya," which are marijuana leaves after their pods have been removed. The word may be derived from potacion de guaya, a potation (from the Latin potere, "to drink") that causes guaya, "lamentation" in Latin American Spanish.

Potency - Usually refers to the THC content in MMJ.

Prescription - A written direction for a therapeutic or corrective agent, specifically: one for the preparation and use of a medicine.

Psychoactive - Drugs that affect the mind or behavior.

Purity - The proportion of active constituent (THC) in a product. For most medical marijuana users, it often refers to the absence of additives such as pesticides and other chemicals.

Reciprocity – Agreement between some states that permits MMID holders to purchase MMJ in certain states outside of their residence. At present, the following states have reciprocity: Arizona, Delaware, Maine, Michigan, Montana and Rhode Island.

Referendum - The principle or practice of submitting to popular vote a measure passed upon or proposed by a legislative body or by popular initiative.

Referring Physician - The doctor who recommends the use of medical marijuana to a patient.

Rescheduling - Moving a drug from one of the five classifications of controlled substances to another. Medical Marijuana advocates desire that marijuana be *rescheduled* from its current position on Schedule I to a lesser-controlled Schedule II or Schedule III.

Rolling tips – Stiff paper used as an inhibitor/filter on a joint. Available at most stores that sell cigarettes.

Sativa - Sativa marijuana is recognized by its size, usually growing up to 8-12 feet tall with long thin leaves. Sativa strains of marijuana are known to emit a sweet smell as they reach maturity. The smoke produced these types of marijuana is generally more mild and lighter with a fruity flavorful taste. The medicinal effects of sativa strains are much more cerebral compared to indica strains. Medical marijuana patients tend to use sativa dominant stains during the daytime because of their energetic and uplifting effects. Sativas are also helpful for treating chronic pain and general stress without the heavy sedation of an indica. Many patients that use medical marijuana throughout the course of a day utilize sativa dominant strains of cannabis to avoid the burnout feeling.

Scale - Marijuana measurement device used to weigh out grams or ounces of marijuana.

Shisha - A mixture of tobacco, molasses, fruit and flavor extracts which is usually smoked in a hookah.

Shwag - Also known as low-grade street marijuana.

Sinsemilla - The Spanish word for "seedless." The highest potency of herbal cannabis comprising the flowering tops of unfertilized female plants.

Skunk - Herbal cannabis with a characteristic odor that is similar to the smell of the skunk animal. Skunk may have a high potency.

Slider – The stem of a bong which contains the bowl. Once the bong is filled with smoke, you "slide" the slider out in order to clear the bong.

Splash guard – A piece inserted into a bong tube to prevent bong water from splashing back into the smoker's mouth.

Spliff – A joint of a mixture of weed and tobacco rolled in a paper.

Stacking – Smoking a different strain of MMJ (or hash) with each hit. This can intensify your high.

Stepping Stone - The theory that experimenting with one drug will naturally lead the person to try other, more harmful drugs.

Strain - A group of plants with a presumed common ancestry with clear-cut physiological but usually not morphological distinctions. Cannabis strains are often referred to as pure indica, mostly indica, indica/sativa, mostly sativa, or pure sativa. Growers or distributors might use other names.

Super Charged – MMJ bud that is tumbled with kief to make it stronger. After treatment, the MMJ is still identified by its strain (e.g., Bubba Kush Super Charged).

Tenon – The part of a tobacco pipe that connects the stem to the bowl.

THC - The active chemical in the compound known as tetrahydrocannabinol. The main psychoactive component of cannabis, and is produced in glandular trichomes, particularly in the unfertilized female flowering tops of the plant.

Tincture - An amber to dark green colored liquid that has been used to melt the THC crystals off marijuana even after the MMJ has been used in a vaporizer. A tincture is usually put under the tongue, where it is absorbed into the body.

Titrate - Determining the strength of a solution or the concentration of a substance in solution in terms of the smallest amount of a reagent of known concentration required to bring about a given effect in reaction with a known volume of the test solution. In medical marijuana, this refers to how much one can smoke/consume in order to produce the first desired effects.

Toke – To take a drag or puff of a marijuana joint/spliff. Also referred to as "blazing."

Tongue bite – A sour, alkaline, burning sensation in the mouth or throat caused by smoking a pipe packed too loosely and/or inhaling too quickly.

Toxicity - Relating to, or caused by a poison or toxin. A substance in small doses may not be harmful, but large doses can produce toxicity in the body.

Trace Elements - The smaller nutrients needed for a healthy marijuana plant growth.

Trichomes - Marijuana plants have large concentrations of cannabinoids in the trichomes. Trichomes on plants are epidermal outgrowths of various kinds. A common type of trichome is a hair. Plant hairs may be unicellular or multicellular, branched or unbranched. Multicellular hairs may have one or several layers of cells. Branched hairs can bedendritic (tree-like), tufted, or stellate (star-shaped). When referring to cannabis specifically, trichomes are the tiny mushroom-shaped appendages covering the buds. The trichomes increase in number as the plant matures. The color of the trichome's head changes as well and indicates the degree of potency. Flowers that are covered in trichomes are typically a "frosty" color and can literally glisten.

Vaporizer – A smoking device used to avoid irritating respiratory toxins in marijuana smoke by heating cannabis to a temperature where the psychoactive ingredients evaporate without causing combustion to carcinogens. You inhale a mist instead of actual smoke, which is proposed to be healthier for the user's lungs than smoking through a pipe.

Wand – A usually glass tube with a wire mesh screen inside used for vaporizing. MMJ is place in the wand (on top the screen) then the open end of the wand is positioned against the heating element of a vaporizer.

Water pipe – A smoking apparatus, as a hookah or narghile, in which the smoke is drawn through a container of water and cooled before reaching the mouth.

Bibliography

Barnes, D., Smith, D., Gatchel, R. J., & Mayer, T. G. (1989). Psychosocioeconomic predictors of treatment success/failure in chronic low-back pain patients. *Spine, 14*, 427-430.

Bumgartner, A., MMJ and Disposable Lighters. Retrieved 6Jan12 from http://www.cannlabs.com/papers/MMJ%20and%20Disposable%20Lighters.pdf

Berman, B. M. & Swyers, J. P. (1999). Complementary medicine treatments for fibromyalgia syndrome. *Best Practices and Research in Clinical Rheumatology, 13*(3), 487-492.

Bigos, S. J., Battie, M. C., & Spengler, D. M. (1991). A prospective study of work perceptions and psychosocial factors affecting the report of back injury. *Spine, 16*, 1-6.

Bingel, U., Rose, M., Gläscher, J., & Büchel, C. (2007). fMRI reveals how pain modulates visual object processing in the ventral visual stream. *Neuron, 55*, 157-167-168.

Bongers, P. M., deWinter, C. R., Kompier, M. A., & Hildebrandt, V. H. (1993). Psychosocial factors at work and musculoskeletal disease. *Scandinavian Journal of Work and Environment Health, 19*(5), 297-312.

Brandstadt, G. (1995). *Chronic pain and anxiety management* (rev. ed.). Victoria, BC, Canada: Niagara House.

Brink, N. E. (1989). The power struggle of workers' compensation–strategies for intervention. *Journal of Applied Rehabilitation Counseling, 20*(1), 25-28.

Burdorf, A., Rossignol, M., Fathallah, F.A., Snook, S. H., & Herrick, R.F. (1997). Challenges in assessing risk factors in epidemiologic studies on back disorders. *American Journal of Industrial Medicine, 32*(2), 143-152.

Cannon, W. B. (1929). *Bodily changes in pain, hunger, fear, and rage.* New York: Appleton-Century-Crofts.

Carter, L. E., McNeil, D. W., Vowles, K. E., Sorrell, J. T., Turk, C. L., & Ries, B. J. (2002). Effects of emotion on pain reports, tolerance and physiology. *Pain Research Management, 7,* 21-30.

Chapman, C.R. & Bonica, J.J. (1985). *Chronic pain.* Kalamazoo: Upjohn.

Chapman, C. R. & Stillman, M. (1996). Pathological pain. In L. Kruger (Ed.), *Pain and touch* (2nd ed.) (pp. 315-42). New York: Academic Press.

Commission on Accreditation of Rehabilitation Facilities. (1995). *Standards manual and interpretive guidelines for medical rehabilitation.* Tuscan, AZ: Author.

Cooper, C. L. & Marshall, J. (1976). Occupational sources of stress: A review of literature relating to coronary heart disease and mental ill health. *Journal of Occupational Psychology, 49,* 11-28.

Corey, D. (1993). *Pain: Learning to live without it.* Toronto: Macmillan Canada.

Crook, J., Tunks, E., Rideout, E., & Brown, G. (1986). Epidemiologic comparison of persistent pain sufferers in a specialty pain clinic and in the community. *Archives of Physical Medicine and Rehabilitation, 67,* 451-455.

D'Arcy, Y. (2006). Treatment strategies for low back pain relief. *Nurse Practitioner, 31*(4), 16-25.

Deardorf, W. W., Rubin, H. S., & Scott, D. W. (1991). Comprehensive multidisciplinary treatment of chronic pain: A follow-up study of treated and non-treated groups. *Pain, 45,* 35-43.

Debruyne, D. , Abessard, F., Bigot, M.C., & Moulin, M. (1994). Comparison of three advanced chromatographic techniques for cannabis identification. United Nations Office and Drugs and Crime, 109-121. Retrieved 6Jan12 from http://www.unodc.org/unodc/en/data-and-analysis/bulletin/bulletin_1994-01-01_2_page009.html#s0001

Deyo, R. A. (1996). Low back pain: A primary care challenge. *Spine, 21*(24), 2826-2832.

Disorbio, J. M. Psychological factors related to pain. *The National Pain Foundation*. Retrieved June 17, 2001, from http://www.painconnection.org

Egan, K. J. & Katon, W. J. (1987). Responses to illness and health in chronic pain patients and healthy adults. *Psychosomatic Medicine, 49*, 470-481.

Ehrlich, G. E. (2003). Low back pain. *Bulletin of the World Health Organization, 81*(9), 671-676.

Fishbain, D. A., Goldberg, M., Meagher, B. R., & Rosomoff, H. (1986). Male and female chronic pain patients categorized by DSM-III psychiatric diagnostic criteria. *Pain, 26*, 181-197.

Flor, H. & Birbaumer, N. (1994). Acquisition of chronic pain; Psychophysiological mechanisms. *American Pain Society Journal, 3*(3), 119-127.

Forgas, J. P. (1998). On being happy and mistaken: Mood effects on the fundamental attribution error. *Journal of Personality and Social Psychology, 75*(2), 318-331.

Fredrickson, B. E.; Trief, P. M., VanBeveren, P., Yuan, H. A., & Baum, G. (1988). Rehabilitation of the patient with chronic back pain: A search for outcome predictors. *Spine, 13*(3), 351-353.

Gallagher, R. M., Rauh, V., Haugh, L. D., Milhous, R., Callas, P. W., Regis, L., et al. (1995). Determinants of return to work among chronic low-back pain patients. *Pain, 39*, 55-67.

Garcy, P., Mayer, T., & Gatchel, R. J. (1996). Recurrent or new injury outcomes after return to work in chronic disabling spinal disorders. *Spine*, *21*(8), 952-959.

Gatchel, R. J., Polatin, P. B., & Mayer, T. G. (1995). The dominant role of psychosocial risk factors in the development of chronic low back pain disability. *Spine*, *20*(24), 2702-2709.

Gatchel, R.J. & Turk, D.C. (1999). Interdisciplinary treatment of chronic pain patients. In R.J. Gatchel & D.C. Turk (eds.). *Psychosocial Factors in Pain: Critical Perspectives* (pp. 435-444). New York: Guilford Publications, Inc.

Gauer, J. (planned 2012). Pain at Work: The Invisible Epidemic of Chronic Pain in America…and What We Can Do to Keep Talent in the Workplace. Colorado Springs: Work-Playground Press.

Gauer, J. (2011). Work Can Be a Playground, Not a Prison (Professional Edition): Creating Positive Growth in your Physical and Emotional Work Environment. Colorado Springs: Work-Playground Press.

Gauer, J. (2011). Work Can Be a Playground, Not a Prison (Basic Edition): How to Make Work Fun Again. Colorado Springs: Work-Playground Press.

Gauer, J. (2009). Fibromyalgia in the workplace: Exploring the impact of chronic pain upon white-collar workers. *Dissertation Abstracts International* (UMI No. 3344894).

Gauer, J. (2006). "How does diversity influence workplace profitability?" Presented at the Institute of Behavior and Applied Management's (IBAM) annual meeting in Memphis in October, 2006.

Gauer, J. (2006). "Stigma and Inclusion of Handicapped People in the Workplace" Presented at the Institute of Behavior and Applied Management's (IBAM) annual meeting in Memphis in October, 2006.

Gauer, J. & Dykman, C. (2005). "Stumbling blocks or stepping stones? Recognizing and overcoming barriers to e-collaboration in communities of practice." *OR Insight, 18*:4, Oct.-Dec.

Gentry, W. D. (1982). Chronic back pain: Does elective surgery benefit patients with evidence of psychological disturbance? *Southern Medical Journal, 75*(10), 1169-1170.

Gilson, I. & Busalacchi, M. (1998). Marijuana for intractable hiccups. *The Lancet, Vol. 351*, January 24, 1998, p. 267

Goldberg, R. T. (1974). Adjustment of children with invisible and visible handicaps: Congenital heart disease and facial burns. *Journal of Counseling Psychology, 21*, 428-432.

Goldstein, D. S. (1995). *Stress, catecholamines, and cardiovascular disease*. New York: Oxford University Press.

Government Statistical Service (GSS) (1998). *The prevalence of back pain in Great Britain in 1998*. London: TSO.

Grotenhermen, Franjo. *Pharmacokinetics and Pharmacodynamics of Cannabinoids* Clin Pharmacokinet 2003; 42 (4): 327-360.

Guest, G. H. & Drummond, P. D. (1992). Effect of compensation on emotional state and disability in chronic back pain. *Pain, 48*, 125-130.

Hadler, N. M. (1996). If you have to prove you are ill, you can't get well. *Spine, 21*, 2397-2400.

Hadler, N. M. (1999). *Occupational musculoskeletal disorders* (2nd ed.) Philadelphia: Lippincott, Williams & Wilkins.

Harrison, R. V. (1978). Person-environment fit and job stress. In C. L. Cooper & R. Payne (Eds.), *Stress at work* (pp. 175-205). Chichester, NY: John Wiley & Sons.

Hazard, R. G., Bendix. A., & Fenwick, J. W. (1991). Disability exaggeration as a predictor of functional restoration outcomes for patients with chronic low back pain. *Spine, 16*(9), 1062-1067.

Hildebrandt, J., Pfingsten, M. Saur, P., & Jansen, J. (1997). Prediction of success from a multidisciplinary treatment program for chronic low back pain. *Spine, 22*(9), 990-1101.

International Association for the Study of Pain (1986). Classification of chronic pain. *Pain, 3*, S1-226.

Izzo, A., Borrelli, F., Capasso, R., DiMarzo, V. & Mechoulam, R. (2009). Non-psychotropic plant cannabinoids: new therapeutic opportunities from an ancient herb. *Trends in Pharmacological Sciences, 30*(10), 515-527.

Karasek, R. (1979). Job demands, job decision latitude, and mental strain: Implications for job redesign. *Administration Science Quarterly, 24*, 285-308.

Keel, P. J. (1984). Psychosocial criteria for patient selection: Review of studies and concepts for understanding chronic back pain. *Neurosurgery, 15*(6), 935-941.

Kerns, R. D., Turk, D. C., & Rudy, T. E. (1985) The West Haven-Yale multidimensional pain inventory. *Pain, 23*, 345-356.

Khalsa, D. & Stauth, C. (1999). *The pain cure.* New York: Warner Books.

Krause, N. & Ragland, D. R. (1994). Occupational disability due to low back pain: A new interdisciplinary classification based on a phase model of disability. *Spine, 19*(9), 1011-1020.

Levine, R. L. (1983). Oxidative modification of glutamine synthetase. I. Inactivation is due to loss of one histidine residue. *Journal of Biological Chemistry, 258*, 11823–11827.

Levy, L. (1972). *Stress and distress in response to psychosocial stimuli.* NY: Pergamon Press.

Limbert, J. (2002, October). *Problems associated with chronic pain claims: Turning the medical perspective into legal evidence.* Paper presented at the Western Forum on Litigating Disability Claims, Vancouver, BC, Canada.

Lindstrom, I., Ohlund, C., Eek, C., Wallin, E., Peterson, L. E., & Nachemson, A. (1992). Mobility, strength, and fitness after a graded activity program for patients with sub-acute low back pain: A randomized prospective clinical study with behavioral therapy approach. *Spine, 17*, 641-652.

Love, A.W. & Peck, C. L. (1987). The MMPI and psychological factors in chronic low back pain: A review. *Pain, 28*, 1-12.

Mayer, T. & Gatchel, R. (1988). *Functional restoration for spinal disorders: The sports medicine approach*. Philadelphia: Lea & Febiger.

McCreary, C., Turner, J., & Dawson, E. (1981). Principal dimensions of the pain experience and psychological disturbance in chronic low back pain patients. *Pain, 11*, 85-92.

Mechoulam R, Peters M, Murillo-Rodriguez E, Hanuš LO (August 2007). Cannabidiol--recent advances. *Chemistry & Biodiversity, 4* (8): 1678–92.

Melzack, R. & Wall, P. D. (1982). *The challenge of pain*. London: Penguin.

Morgan, C.J., Curran, H.V. (2008). Effects of cannabidiol on schizophrenia-like symptoms in people who use cannabis. *The British Journal of Psychiatry :The Journal of Mental Science, 192* (4): 306–7.

Minton, E. (1994, July). Implementing a can-do attitude. *Hemisphere*, 31.

Mundy, R. R., Moore, S. C., Corey, J. B., & Mundy, G. D. (1994). Disability syndrome: The effects of early vs. delayed rehabilitation intervention. *American Association of Occupational Health Nurses (AAOHN) Journal, 42*(8), 379-383.

Nicholas, M. K., Wilson, P. H., & Goyen, J. (1992). Comparison of cognitive-behavioral group treatment and an alternative non- psychological treatment for chronic low back pain. *Pain, 48*, 339-347.

Nutt, D., King, L. A., Saulsbury, W., & Blakemore, C. (2007). Development of a rational scale to assess the harm of drugs of potential misuse. *The Lancet 369* (9566): 1047–1053.

Okifuji, A., Turk, D. C., & Kalauokalani, D. (1999). Clinical outcome and economic evaluation of multidisciplinary pain centers. In A.R. Bock, E.F. Kremer, & E. Fernandez (Eds.), *Handbook of pain syndromes: Biopsychosocial perspectives* (pp. 77-97). Mahwah, NJ: Lawrence Erlbaum Associates.

Ron de Kloet, E., Joels, M., & Holsboer, F. (2005). Stress and the brain: from adaptation to disease. *Nature Reviews Neuroscience 6* (6): 463–475.

Russo, C. M. & Brose, W. G. (1998). Chronic pain. *Annual Review of Medicine, 49*, 123-133.

Sanders, S. J., Rucker, K. S., Anderson, K. O., Harden, R. N., Jackson, K. W., & Vicente, P. J. (1995). Clinical practice guidelines for chronic non-malignant pain syndrome patients. *Journal of Back and Musculoskeletal Rehabilitation, 5*, 115-120.

Sarno, J. E. (1991). *Healing back pain: The mind-body connection.* New York: Warner.

Selye, H. (1936). A syndrome produced by diverse nocuous agents. *Nature, 138*, 32.

Selye, H. (1956). *The stress of life.* New York: McGraw-Hill.

Selye, H. (1975). Confusion and controversy in the stress field. *Journal of Human Stress 1*: 37–44.

Smith, B. (2000). Chronic pain initiative: Report of the Chair of the Chronic Pain Panels for the Ontario Workplace Safety and Insurance Board: Ontario Canada.

Smith, M. J. & Sainfort, P. C. (1989). A balance theory of job design for stress reduction. *International Journal of Industrial Ergonomics, 4*, 67-79.

Sorenson, J., Bengtsson, A., Backman, E., Henriksson, K. G., & Bengtsson, M. (1995). Pain analysis in patients with fibromyalgia: Effects of intravenous morphine, lidocaine, and ketamine. *Scandinavian Journal of Rheumatology, 24*(3), 360-365.

Spitzer, W. O., LeBlanc, F .E., & Dupuis, M. (1987). Scientific approach to the assessment and management of activity-related spinal disorders. A monograph for clinicians. Report of the Quebec Task Force on Spinal Disorders. *Spine, 12*, S5-59.

Strang, J.P. (1985). In G.M. Aronoff (Ed.), *The Chronic Disability Syndrome, Evaluation and Treatment of Chronic Pain,* pp. 247-58. Baltimore, Maryland: Urban & Schwarzenberg.

Tan, S. Y. (1982). Cognitive and cognitive-behavioral methods for pain control: A selective review. *Pain, 12*, 201-228.

Thomas, A., Stevenson, L.A., Wease, K.M., Price, M.R., Baillie, G., Ross, R.A., & Pertwee, R.G. (2005). Evidence that the plant cannabinoid Δ^9-tetrahydrocannabivarin is a cannabinoid CB_1 and CB_2 receptor antagonist. *British Journal of Pharmacology, 146*(7), 917-925.

Tollison, D., Kriegel, M. A., & Downie, G. R. (1985). Chronic low back pain: Results of treatment at the pain therapy center. *Southern Medical Journal, 78*(11), 1291-1295.

Turk, D. C. (1996). Biopsychosocial perspective on chronic pain. In R. J. Gatchel & D. C. Turk (Eds.), *Psychological approaches to pain management: A practitioner's handbook* (pp. 3-32). New York: Guilford Press.

Turner, J. A. & Chapman, C. R. (1982). Psychological interventions for chronic pain: A critical review. II: Operant conditioning, hypnosis, and cognitive-behavioral therapy. *Pain, 12*, 23-46.

Turner, J. A. & Romano, J. M. (1990). Psychologic and psychosocial evaluation. In J. J. Bonica (Ed.), *The management of pain: Vol. I.* (2nd ed.; pp. 595-609). Philadelphia: Lea & Febiger.

Ursin, H., Murison, R., & Knardahl, S. (1983). Conclusion: Sustained activation and disease. In H. Ursin & R. Murison (Eds.), *Biological and psychological basis of psychosomatic disease* (pp. 269-277). Oxford: Pergamon Press.

Volkmann, H., Norregaard, J., Jacobsen, S., Danneskiold-Samsoe, B., Knoke, G., & Nehrdich, D. (1997). Double-blind, placebo-controlled cross-over study of intravenous S-adenosyl-L-methionine in patients with fibromyalgia. *Scandinavian Journal of Rheumatology, 26*(3), 206-211.

Waddell, G. (1992). Biopsychosocial analysis of low back pain. In M. Nordin & T. L. Visher (Eds.), *Bailliere's clinical rheumatology. Common low back pain: Prevention of chronicity* (pp. 523-557). London: Bailliere Tindall.

Waddell, G., Sommerville, D., Henderson, I., Newton, M., & Main, C. J. (1993). A fear avoidance beliefs questionnaire (FABQ) and the role of fear avoidance beliefs in chronic low back pain and disability. *Pain, 52,* 157-168.

Watson, L. A. (1999). "Mirror, mirror on the wall…": An exploratory study of physical disability and women's expressed body image. *Dissertation Abstracts International, 59* (9), 5173B (UMI No. 9904366).

End Notes

[1] Kepple & Freisthler, 2012
[2] Nutt, King, Saulsbury, & Blakemore, 2007
[3] Retrieved 27Aug12 from: http://medicalmarijuana.procon.org/view.background-resource.php?resourceID=865
[4] http://en.wikipedia.org/wiki/Marijuana. Retrieved 18Oct11
[5] http://www.tokeofthetown.com/2012/02/oregon_issues_medical_marijuana_cards_to_out-of-st.php
[6] http://www.thetimes.co.uk
[7] http://ireadculture.com/2011/08/news/marijuana-patient-statistics/ Retrieved 12Oct11. Original source: *The Coloradoan*
[8] http://www.cdphe.state.co.us/hs/medicalmarijuana/statistics.html
[9] Retrieved 13Nov12 from http://www.kval.com/news/health/Medical-marijuana-group-buds-with-Oregons-new-top-cop-168072676.html
[10] "US medical cannabis policy eased". *BBC News*. 20 October 2009. http://news.bbc.co.uk/2/hi/8315603.stm. Retrieved 30 October 2009
[11] http://mlis.state.md.us/2011rs/billfile/SB0308.htm. Retrieved 2Sept11
[12] http://norml.org/index.cfm?Group_ID=3391. Retrieved 2Sept11
[13] "Employers now able to fire medical marijuana users legally in Washington". MedicalMarijuanaBill.com. 13-06-2011. http://medicalmarijuanabill.com/2011/06/employers-fire-legally-washington/. Retrieved 31-07-2011
[14] Corey-Bloom, et al., 2012
[15] Retrieved 27Aug12 from: http://medicalmarijuana.procon.org/view.additional-resource.php?resourceID=000191
[16] Mechoulam, Peters, Murillo-Rodriguez, & Hanuš, 2007
[17] Morgan & Curran, 2008
[18] From http://en.wikipedia.org/wiki/Cannabinoid#Types. Retrieved 6Jan12.
[19] Thomas, Stevenson, Wease, Price, Baillie, Ross, & Pertwee, 2005
[20] Full Spectrum Labs
[21] Debruyne, Abessard, Bigot, & Moulin, 1994
[22] Full Spectrum Labs, CannLabs
[23] Gilson & Busalacchi, 1998
[24] http://www.cdphe.state.co.us/hs/medicalmarijuana/statistics.html

[25] Gatchel & Turk, 1999
[26] Khalsa & Stauth, 1999
[27] Deyo, 1996; Snook, 2005
[28] Chapman & Bonica, 1985; Strang, 1985
[29] Bingel, Rose, Gläscher & Büchel, 2007
[30] Mayer & Gatchel, 1988
[31] Limbert, 2002
[32] Goldberg, 1974; Watson, 1999
[33] Sarno, 1991
[34] Ehrlich, 2003
[35] Gauer, 2009
[36] Sanders et al., 1995
[37] Sanders et al., 1995
[38] Ehrlich, 2003
[39] Smith, 2000
[40] Bigos, Battie, & Spengler, 1994; Spitzer, LeBlanc, & Dupuis, 1987
[41] Deyo, 1996
[42] Ehrlich, 2003
[43] Disorbio, 2001
[44] Bingel, Rose, Gläscher, and Büchel, 2007
[45] Deardorf et al., 1991
[46] Ehrlich, 2003
[47] Hadler, 1996
[48] Ehrlich, 2003, p. 674
[49] Commission on Accreditation of Rehabilitation Facilities, 1995; Hadler, 1999; Russo & Brose, 1998
[50] IASP, 1986, p. 1
[51] Smith, 2000, p. 15
[52] Flor & Birgaumer, 1994; IASP, 1986; Russo & Brose, 1998
[53] Khalsa and Stauth, 1999, p. 20
[54] Flor & Birbaumer, 1994
[55] Chapman and Stillman, 1996
[56] Smith, 2000
[57] D'Arcy, 2006
[58] Waddell, Sommerville, Henderson, Newton & Main, 1993
[59] Brink, 1989
[60] Mundy, Moore, Corey, & Mundy, 1994

[61] Deyo, 1996
[62] Ehrlich, 2003, p. 671
[63] Mayer and Gatchel, 1988
[64] Government Statistical Service [GSS], 1998
[65] Barnes, Smith, Gatchel, & Mayer, 1989; Smith, Bigos et al., 1991; Garcy et al., 1996; Gatchel & Mayer, 1989; Gatchel, Polatin, & Mayer, 1995; Hazard, Bendix, & Fenwick, 1991; Hildebrandt, Pfingsten, Saur, & Jansen, 1997; Lindstrom et al., 1992; Okifuji, Turk, & Kalauokalani, 1999; Turk, 1996a
[66] Cooper & Marshall, 1976; Levy, 1972; Selye, 1936; Smith & Sainfort, 1989
[67] Cannon, 1929
[68] Berman & Swyers, 1999
[69] Guest & Drummond, 1992
[70] Ehrlich, 2003
[71] Sorensen, Bengtsson, Backman, Henriksson, & Bengtsson, 1995; Volkmann et al., 1997
[72] Selye, 1975.
[73] Ron de Kloet, Joels, & Holsboer, 2005
[74] Cannon, 1929
[75] Selye, 1956
[76] Goldstein, 1995; Levine, 1983; Ursin, Murison & Knardahl, 1983
[77] Harrison, 1978
[78] Karasek, 1979
[79] Waddell, 1992
[80] Brandstadt, 1995; Carter et al., 2002; Corey, 1993; Forgas, 1998
[81] Melzack and Wall, 1982
[82] Krause & Ragland, 1994; Gallagher et al., 1995
[83] Turk, 1996a
[84] Bongers, deWinter, Kompier, and Hilebrandt, 1993
[85] Burdorf, Rossignol, Fathallah, Snook, and Herrick, 1997
[86] Disorbio, 2001
[87] Russo & Brose, 1998
[88] Carter et al., 2002
[89] Gallagher et al., 1995; Krause & Ragland, 1994
[90] Nicholas, Wilson & Goyen, 1992; Tan, 1982
[91] Crook, Tunks, Rideout, & Brown, 1986; Egan & Katon, 1987; Fishbain, Goldberg, Meagher, Steele, & Rosomoff, 1986; Fredrikson et al., 1988; Gentry, 1982; Keel, 1984; Kerns, Turk, & Rudy, 1985; Love & Peck, 1987; McCreary,

Turner, & Dawson, 1981; Tollison, 1989; Turner & Chapman, 1982; Turner & Romano, 1990

[92] Grotenhermen, 2003

[93] From http://www.wikihow.com/Use-a-Water-Bong. Retrieved 12Sept11. Reprinted under creative common license.

[94] From http://weedsmokersguide.com/anatomy-hookah-pipe. Retrieved 15Sept11

[95] From http://nlnaturalrx.com/edibles. Retrieved 2Nov11 and reprinted with permission.

[96] Bumgartner, 2012

[97] From http://www.wikihow.com/Use-a-Water-Bong. Retrieved 12Sept11. Reprinted under creative common license.

Appendix

Pain Information Resources

American Academy of Pain Management (www.aapainmanage.org) – Informational pages, medical topics, an on-line pain management community, newsletters, and access to current research on pain management.

American Chronic Pain Association (www.theacpa.org) - Offers support and information. Also see North American Chronic Pain Association of Canada (www.chronicpaincanada.org).

American Pain Foundation (www.painfoundation.org) - This site contains vast links for patient information, advocacy, and media resources.

American Society of Anesthesiologists (www.asahq.org) - Explains the definition, history, and scope of anesthesiology, as well as addressing issues such as patient safety.

Beth Israel Medical Center Department of Pain Medicine and Palliative Care (www.stoppain.org) - This site includes downloadable PowerPoint® modules and an on-line *Pain Multimedia Library*.

CFIDS Association of America (www.cfids.org) - Addresses symptoms, diagnosis, and treatment of Chronic Fatigue and Immune Dysfunction Syndrome.

International Association for the Study of Pain® (www.iasp-pain.org) - Mainly geared toward health professionals, this site's *subject index* contains numerous newsletters and in-depth articles.

Mayday Pain Project at City of Hope Hospital (www.may.coh.org) – Provides information on everything from occupational pain to hospitals and therapy.

National Headache Foundation (www.headaches.org) - Discusses headache symptoms, medications, and treatments.

National Institute of Neurological Disorders and Stroke (www.ninds.nih.gov/health_and_medical/disorders/chronic_pain.htm) - This *chronic pain information page* discusses treatments, prognoses, organizations, and research.

National Pain Foundation (www.painconnection.org) - Provides information about symptoms, treatment options, and support programs for patients and their families.

Occupational Safety and Health Administration (www.osha.gov) - Provides regulatory compliance information (by industry) regarding worker safety and health.

National Institute for Occupational Safety and Health (www.cdc.gov/niosh) - Conducts research and makes recommendations for the prevention of work-related illness, stress, and injury.

Pain.com (http://pain.com) - This site covers a multitude of pain categories, as well as interviews and full-length articles by noted pain professionals.

Pain & The Law (www.painandthelaw.org) – A guide to statues, regulations, entitlement programs, agencies, and organizations.

WebMD® (www.webmd.com) - Search by topics such as occupational, acute, and chronic pain.

Your Orthopaedic Connection (www.orthoinfo.aaos.org) - Takes you to sites dedicated to problems of the neck, shoulder, arm/elbow, spine, hand, hip, knee, and foot/leg.

Subject Index

Alcohol 10, 16
    For cleaning 83-85, 87

Blunt 95, 101

Bong 64, 66-67, 90, 95, 97, 102-104, 106
    How to smoke 68
    Tips 83-84

Bubbler 64, 67, 96

Cannabinoids 20-23, 50-51, 96, 100, 108
    Properties 20-23
    Receptors 15, 98

Cannabis Indica 49, 52-54, 78, 87, 97, 99, 101, 106-108

Cannabis Sativa 49, 52-54, 78, 97, 100-102, 106-107

Caviar 53-55, 98
    Also see *Infusion*

Dispensary 10, 12-13, 21, 44-45, 49-50, 52-58, 77-78, 95, 98-101, 103
    Choosing 49-50

Enhanced bud 53, 55, 99
    See *Infusion*

Flushing 55-56, 100

Financial assistance programs 45
    Coloradans 4 Cannabis 45
    Medical Marijuana Assistance Program of America 45

Hashish (hash) 52-53, 75-76, 80-81, 85, 87, 95, 97-100, 102, 104, 106

Headache 17, 54-56, 120

Hookah 64, 69-72, 101, 106, 108
    How to smoke 72

Hybrid 52, 101

Indica
    See *Cannabis Indica*

Infused flower 53, 55, 102
    See *Infusion*

Infusion 53-55, 98, 102

Joint 42, 54-60, 76, 78-79, 81, 86, 95, 98, 100-102, 104-107
   Rolling by hand 57-58
   Rolling with cigarette machine 58-59

Kief 53, 81, 98-99, 102, 107

Lighter (butane) 68, 73, 75, 82-84, 86, 90, 106

Limits letter 80, 102,

Marijuana plant (uses) 47-48

Medibles 13, 50, 55, 57, 64, 78, 100, 103

Medical Marijuana Card 10-11, 14, 49, 53, 77, 99, 103

Pain (chronic) 10, 15-16, 18- 20, 23-40, 43-44, 52, 54, 83, 93, 101, 103, 106, 123-124
   Vs. Sleep 38-40
   And Stress 30-37
   Ten Facts 26

Pipe 42, 47, 54-56, 64-70, 74-76, 78, 80-82, 86-92, 96-98, 101, 103-104, 107-108
   Water pipe 64-69, 108
      How to smoke 66
   Glass pipes 64, 70, 72-73, 84, 87, 95, 104, 108
      How to smoke 73
   Wooden pipe 72, 73-76, 78, 87
      How to smoke 75-76
   How to clean 92
   Tips 79-82, 87-92

Reciprocity 11-12, 49, 80, 105

Sativa
   see *Cannabis Sativa*

Sleep 38-40

Shisha 70-72, 106

Storage (MMJ) 51, 78, 87

Super charged bud 53, 55, 107
   See *Infusion*

Tincture 50, 107

Tobacco 19, 52, 56-57, 59, 64, 67, 69-73, 75-76, 79-80, 85, 87-88, 90-92, 98, 102- 107
   Classes 79

Tongue bite 76, 90, 107

Trichomes 54, 100, 102, 107-108

Trip (bad) 20, 42-43, 44

Vaporizer 42, 55-56, 60-64, 69, 76, 78, 85-87, 90, 95, 101-102, 104, 107-108
   How to use 62
   Replacing the screen 63
   Tips 85-86
   How to clean 85-86
   Portable 86

About the Author

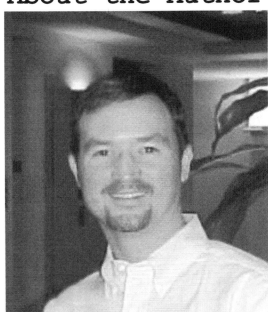

For the past two decades, Dr. Gauer has suffered from fibromyalgia, degenerative disc disease, and chronic Lyme disease, but he perseveres each day with his mission to live a productive life and help others. With his own chronic pain influencing his professional careers in management and education, Dr. Gauer has studied and published on the effects of chronic pain among working adults. Based on his in-depth research and first-hand experiences, Jeff brings to the public the first authoritative book with clear and practical advice for those considering smoking medical marijuana (MMJ).

Jeff has been a professional musician; a full-time foreign missionary; an international sales and marketing executive; and a college instructor. Dr. Gauer also served as a commissioned officer in the US Army Intelligence Corps and is a member of Mensa (The High IQ Society). He holds degrees in English (BA), international business (MBA), and organization and management (Ph.D.). As a manager and educator, Jeff specializes in organizational strategy and invisible disabilities in the workplace.

Dr. Gauer's patented Rest-A-Desk (a reclinable computer workstation – www.restadesk.com) is expected to be available in fall 2013.

Jeff and his daughter reside in the US Midwest.

My Notes

Made in the USA
Charleston, SC
31 December 2012